"Reading *Sparks From The Heart* did just that, it sparked my heart, leading me inwards to my connection to myself. Narrated from a familiar, gentle, sweet, and joyful tone, Marnie highlights the importance of connecting with and responding to life demands from a heart space, and the physical benefits that follow. I recommend this book for anyone doing their inner child work, or anyone who has a heavy heart, Marnie will soothe it by sharing her journey back to her heart."

- Flow Escolan, Bikram Yoga Teacher

"*Sparks from the Heart* offers a playfully sensuous nudge to anyone who currently finds themselves searching. The author daringly presents readers with an energetic invitation to delve further inwards. To help illuminate the science that is so often enshrouded within spirituality, and consequently, to enable us to become deftly more attune to life as it's happening in this very moment."

- Peter Mulholland, Client and Friend

"Marnie shares her growing in-depth awareness of how the heart and mind, when working in synchronicity, develop wisdom. She has reflected deeply and helps us understand how to work with the new consciousness that is here on the planet now waiting for us to find the wisdom and courage to claim as we reconfigure a planet that nurtures freedom, human rights, and a genuine next-level of wellbeing."

- Ruth Lamb, PhD. Author of *Human Becoming: A Guide to Soul-Centered Living.*

D1499078

Dear. Kim,

Thank you soooo
much for coming out..
Enjoy the book ♥

With love, Marnie.

A Philosophical Journey of the Soul's
Incarnation into Your Subtle Heart

Sparks
from the
Heart

MARNIE O'FARRELL

This book is dedicated to my fellow sisters, and to the lineage of the rose. May the divine feminine return, may you feel welcomed, may you feel safe, and may you be successful in sharing your gifts in their fullness.

To all beings who are searching for their own sacred heart, know that Christ consciousness was here on this planet before religion was created. Although it can be a part of religion too, it doesn't have borders or any one particular expression in its outward form. You could be wearing stilettos, rubber boots, or no shoes at all. You could be dark skinned or light skinned, man, woman, or any gender, tall or short, have all your teeth or none— none of that really matters. Christ consciousness in human form, grows forth from the cultivation of goodness from the inside out, and although it will ask you to clean house of all which is not that, it has no prerequisites other than an open and willing heart.

To Mother earth, may we all feel the unconditional love that you have for us, your children.

May we all remember.

"The love that you withold is
the pain that you carry."

~Ralph Waldo Emerson

Contents

Preface

Sparks from the Heart: A Philosophical Journey of the Soul's Incarnation into Your Subtle Heart is my first book. Writing it felt like being in a thrilling new relationship, while also being pregnant with an energetic child—an exciting and uncomfortable combination. The *Sparks from the Heart* experience took me where I needed to go, to what I needed to see, and into the perspective I needed to observe, allowing me to bring through the lessons that would make this book what it was intended to be. There was a dance I entered when writing this that took my fullness for life, internalized it, and had it stream out through lines of gold energy from the tips of my fingers. It was a process that required me to be slow and steady, and truly focused.

At first, I thought I was writing this book to teach others about the basics of energy healing, the energetics of Alzheimer's, and how to understand illness in a more holistic way. Not surprisingly, *Sparks from the Heart* has become that plus so much more. In the wake after all the global changes that happened in 2020, writing this book became a deep and well-traveled journey. I spent more time with myself than ever before, and fittingly so, as Alzheimer's teaches us to remember more fully who we are.

What I hope you take from this book is a perspective that lightens you, gives you new knowledge into the nature of the human heart and the human spirit, and creates more opportunities for joy, connection, and empowerment in your life. It's been a gift for me to share my heart with you in these pages, and for that, I'm grateful.

Introduction

Welcome Dear, I am elated that you've decided to join me. This book is about Alzheimer's disease and another intrinsic part of our health which is rarely included in the Western medical model—the human soul. I had the experience of working with an Alzheimer's client who was largely non-verbal by the time we met, and since I was unable to get to know her through conversation, my curiosity got the better of me and a book began to take form. It caused me to research the physical diagnosis of Alzheimer's, and it was the first time that I considered bridging the world of energetics with the world of Western medicine.

I discovered that Western medicine understands Alzheimer's to be a neurodegenerative disease, which is caused by the buildup of **β-amyloid plaques** and **neurofibrillary tangles** between and inside neurons in the brain. In Alzheimer's, these naturally occurring proteins accumulate (for reasons seemingly beyond our control) to a level which is toxic for us, and that causes neurons to die in a way that progressively deteriorates different regions of the brain. Neuron death first obstructs the transfer of electrical impulses into the area of the brain that stores new memories, and then as the disease progresses we lose access to our stored memories too.

That is a brief overview of the Western medical model, but this book is written in another language—the language of energy. It's a language which understands that it is consciousness, *the living essence of who we are*, that creates illness into form. Underneath the "woo-woo" packaging that I unwrapped energy healing from years ago, I found a subtle architectural blueprint detailing how the egoic nature of our consciousness interfaces with our physical form. In simpler terms, how the mind, emotion, body, and spirit work together to create what we are living. As energy healing is a relatively unknown yet budding field, I wrote this book for someone to whom this type of information may be new. Alzheimer's disease is conventionally understood as a disease of the mind, so the perspective I share with you here may also be new. That's because this book considers the first manifestation of Alzheimer's disease to be one of the subtle heart.

The human heart at a physical level pumps blood in and pumps blood out, and never stops until we die, and there is a similar truth in the physiology of our subtle heart. We breathe in the world with our breath and through our chakras, and then we breathe it out again. We also don't stop doing this until we die. But more often than not, we forget that to breathe properly, we need to breathe the truth—the realness—of who we are, in and out while we breathe oxygen. Here on earth, it's common that we forget what this deep realness feels like from such a young age that we don't even remember we've forgotten. I was one of those people, and what happens to us is this: we become capable of living from the mind, and we forget the beauty and balance that comes from knowing the depths of our own unique heart.

If you are already familiar with human energetics, you might find an overview of my discoveries fascinating. While if you are not familiar, rest assured that

I am lovingly dedicated to bringing you into my frame of mind. In fact, that's entirely what this book is about.

Overview of my research:

The third eye chakra and the pineal gland it connects into, are in proximity to where the medical world has located the build up of toxic proteins in Alzheimer's research.

The way that the symptoms of Alzheimer's progress is mirrored in the way that the lower three layers of the aura would deteriorate if the soul of that person was no longer fully incarnated into its human vessel.

Experience with my client suggested that her awareness was now living in another density of consciousness; that her soul was travelling.

If you're someone in research mode, you can find a deeper dive into these bullets on the third page of chapter seventeen. On the other hand, if you are someone looking to sink in and soothe your soul with a story, I suggest that you start to read from the beginning. Many times when we are confronted with illness, the roles we are offered to play are ones steeped in some pretty negative emotions. *Sparks from the Heart* will not offer you another one of those roles. Instead, this book is dosed with love, compassion, and curiosity. It offers you the opportunity to play a new leading role as the caretaker of your health in a more empowered way than many of us are used to.

Sparks from the Heart offers a fresh take on ancient wisdom and includes lessons to activate the power of your soul and the alchemical magic that comes with it. My branches of knowledge come from shamanism, enlightenment principles, energy medicine, and the embodied and experiential wisdom from my own life.

This book is written as a big wave that brings you to the undercurrent. Rather than offer you a quick fix to the experience which you may find yourself in, it's about learning the deeper meaning so that we can heal in a way that transforms generations.

The field of energetics is client-centered in its approach, which means that its best medicine comes from the inside out. What that means for you is that *Sparks from the Heart* holds a template, and that you will be the one to fill it. The healing principle that weaves these pages together is available to everyone. It's the alchemical magic of a heart that unifies with what is before it with love, acceptance, and discernment.

Hold space for your curiosity to allow in new possibilities, and take breaths when you need them. I'll even remind you to breathe if you are someone who tends to forget. If you notice that you are skeptical, honor it, and embrace it as a mechanism of self-preservation, which is also natural. Skepticism may pop up from time to time because the story that I share here is one full of the mystical rather than what our traditional society may consider to be real. On the other hand, if this book makes you feel in any way more at ease, more compassion, and more understanding, I smile with you.

I know first-hand that being on earth is not always a walk in the park, and if you are a soul who is experiencing difficulty and pain, this book is intended to be like a friend who has come to offer you a shoulder to lean on. I invite you to curl up somewhere cozy, allow yourself to rest, and consider my words like a humble rose whose beauty is more fully received if you slow down, quiet your thoughts, and take time to breathe in the scent of its essence. As you do this, I hope you get lost in the story. And then, when it's over and when you feel ready, I hope that you sit up straight again with even more joy in your heart. I am certain that you can, and I know that you deserve to live a life where you're standing in the magic of your soul's light.

Chapter One:
The Answer Key

There is a train of thought that compares one physical human incarnation to that of an entire universe. In this philosophy, each human soul is gifted with the opportunity to run their very own personal universe, also known as one human vessel, and bestowed upon them is full sovereignty to live, express, learn, and grow as they please. What these human universes sometimes fail to notice, is how uniquely interwoven they are into the fabric of life around them.

***

Vulnerability comes from expressing the truth of who you are to the outside world, wouldn't you agree? I find myself going back over things . . . as I am now, intending to make my vision as smooth and clear as possible. The voice of an old yoga teacher named Brad pops into my head. It's a lesson. In class, as we laid in dead-body pose (a pose of utter stillness) he'd say, "Once we realize that we are all a little crazy, then we can all just be a little crazy together." True though, isn't it? We are all a little weird on the inside, and life is more fun that way. It's more full and real. I know this to be true, but I'm still learning the wisdom of this lesson.

For the last two years, I have been a multidimensional detective of sorts, and Al has been my focal client.

Multidimensional in this case meaning the dimensions of the mind, body, spirit, and emotions . . . and Al meaning Alzheimer's. For the purposes of this book, Alzheimer's has become more than a diagnosis or a series of symptoms. Al (the dis-ease) has become an integral character in the story, and he (as I have personified him to be) will appear throughout it in more ways than one. Some of his expressions will be mystical while others will be much more literal, and all of them are here as teachers to support you in expanding the relationship that you have with illness.

One day, Al walked into the clinic where I was interning through the soul of a woman named Ms. J, and as I worked with her over a series of months, I realized that he also existed (in a much less physically manifested way), within myself. Alzheimer's is not contagious. What I mean by this is that like attracts like, and that a deep resonance with something usually means that our soul wants us to pay attention to that same aspect in ourselves. When I met Ms. J, a feeling of resonance existed deeply within me, and the investigation that began with her arrival, soon pivoted toward my own internal world.

I'm a Scorpio in this lifetime, so my innate direction is to make my way into the depths, dig deep, and find the pearls buried down in the bottom of the ocean. It has been no different for this assignment. As a metaphysically inclined professional and feminine spirit, I've learned that digging in the darkness can be disorienting and *dark* sometimes, but I never go in empty-handed because I have a tool kit. Inside this tool kit are: my curiosity, my intuition, a personal resonance for pioneering thought, a spiritual heart that has been nurtured and grown over many lifetimes, and a strong connection to the earth and her kingdoms. I also trust deeply that I am never separate from love, no matter how separate I may feel. It's through experience that

I've come to realize the feeling of separateness is natural when we investigate the unknown, and that once we shed light into the dark places we are going, the feeling of loving connection always returns.

Let's not waste any time. I've decided to lead with a bang! This first story is my favorite from when I was in detective mode for *Sparks from the Heart*. It was a phase in my process where I put my faith in the power of my intention and then surrendered it to God. I listened for spiritual guidance and then . . . "let things flow, baby." This phase was all about trusting the experiences I was given, and it was during this time that life led me to the answer key for this book. Was I ever relieved—the flow came through after months of quivering uncertainty. I had decided to write this book before I knew what the story would be, and as far as deep diving goes, my oxygen levels were running perilously low.

The answer key, in case you're wondering, is a healing tool that stems from the understanding of how energy and vibration work in this reality. It's the knowledge that we naturally assimilate new codes of energy all the time: when we read a new book, listen to others talk, or take in new experiences. A piece of esoteric wisdom says that if you really want to heal from something, assistance can come to you through connecting with the vibration of someone who has already healed from the same thing. You just need to find a person who has become intimate with their disease and healed in a holistic way; an individual who has learned their lessons through an inner battle similar to your own. Someone who has taken the hero's journey[1] and is now emanating the answer key.

If you find such a person in your life, what I suggest that you do, in your most polite and curious demeanor, is ask to hang out with them for a little while—to just

1   Joseph Campbell, *The Hero with a Thousand Faces*. New York: Pantheon Books, 1968.

be with them. By sitting beside them and being open to receiving who they are, the healing codes that match your need can be transferred into your aura through the openness you are offering with your curiosity. All you then have to do is integrate those codes for yourself. I make this sound easy, but it requires intelligent and intentional effort and more of your personal energy to be invested in your healing journey.

The good news is if this deeper journey feels right for you, you will know because there will be passion in your heart burning to begin . . . *and to keep reading this book.* Another one of my yoga teachers named Christian now comes to mind and a smile ignites on my face as I hear his voice in my head. Sometimes in class when we were dripping in sweat and feeling lightheaded, he'd say to us, "Nothing good is ever easy," and pose the rhetorical question, "Why else do you keep coming back to the torture chamber?" We would say nothing, but we all knew the answer. It was because inside this self-created pressure and commitment to practice that we were evolving.

Here and now, for whatever reason that you picked up this book, the same truth applies. I'm not going to sugarcoat it, nothing good is ever easy (simple but not easy). True healing means making new choices, evolving outdated habits, and questioning all angles of your perception. However, the hero does get moments of reprieves, and the experience of the answer key should feel as such. While you are meeting with your answer key, little insights may come through. You may have moments of mirroring or reflection, and the ability to ask questions, but mostly the answer key comes through vibration, and that transference is not a part of your conscious awareness. It's like being gifted the vibrational road map to your desired destination, and the way that you read it is to listen to your heart and to hold yourself accountable to walking the path one step at a time. The gift in the answer key is that your inner knowing can now show you the way because the solution has been internalized.

Remember how I mentioned the feeling of separation that comes from diving into the depths of the mystery that is the bottom of the ocean? My deep dive was when I decided with zero hesitation that I was going to write this book, and the events leading up to this spontaneous and unexpected plunge went something like this: it was a beautiful Vancouver summer and I had just graduated from energy healing school on a total high because I had, in my opinion, completely rocked my final presentation. I gave everything I had into my project and spent my time dedicated to the threading together of evidence. It's what happens when passion for a subject and a personal drive to fulfill some inner longing meet. My teachers encouraged me to consider turning what I had written into a book, and I felt very full, reaping the fruits of my work on that fragrant summer's day.

A week later I traveled across Canada, from British Columbia to Ontario, to visit my family, and I was still riding the wave. I spoke enthusiastically and aligned with a publisher in a matter of weeks, by two degrees of separation, and only one town over from where I grew up. The publishing house focused on women's empowerment, health, and well-being. Wouldn't you know it, exactly my professional field. All the ducks had lined up in a row . . . except for one. The Marnie duck. Do you know that age-old saying, "Look before you leap" that's typically paired with a picture of a man about to walk off a cliff? Well, have you ever had a moment in your life where you forget to do that and take a leap forward without even thinking because the momentum you are experiencing makes the leap momentarily invisible? Then you land. You take a look around, and the first words that come to mind are . . . oh shit. Well,

I was having one of those moments, thinking, what have I gotten myself into? The days were dwindling away, I was feeling the stress build up on my shoulders, and nothing was coming through to be written.

Here's another way of putting it. I was at the part of an adventure story where you realize you are lost . . . and then you proceed to step into a big puddle. Your shoes get totally soaked, and when this happens, there is an exact and precise shift in your thoughts. What you had previously registered as exciting and spontaneous, now feels uncomfortable and far from home. The diva in me would have put her hand in the air and said in a quick and sarcastic way, "I'm over this." As far as this book went, that's exactly where my mind was in the moments before meeting Doña María Apaza. I was worried and unsure, but then on a fateful day in mid-November, four days before my thirty-first birthday, something shifted.

I was visiting my friend Megs and her partner in Mount Shasta when the universe aligned in just the nick of time, and I had the unexpected opportunity to sit with a remarkable woman. I was invited to a small gathering near a mountain in California, where I met Doña María. She was a woman nearing her centennial year who was joyfully present in her body; one of those rare and special humans who come around once in a generation. A soul who has attained so much, and having walked through compassion's door, she had chosen to rest in the embodiment of the Divine Mother. Short in stature and missing some teeth, Doña María entered the room with the assistance of her team. I watched her with curiosity, noticing that she needed help to walk and sit down, and that she accepted that help without any sense of it being demeaning. In fact, she seemed to welcome it as part and parcel of aging, and something that had nothing to do with her sense of worth. Her ease came with her ability to trust life, and that ease was expressed through more than just her physicality because there is also energy within and around us; it is life force energy, and it's the same energy that you're learning from when you witness your answer key. It is the energy that makes the difference between a dead body and a living one, and the life force energy in this ninety-eight-year-old lady was still very much alive. Doña María had an effervescent joy that permeated her eyes, her clothes, her voice, and her everything. Her soul was on purpose, and this type of connection is what inspires life in all human vessels.

Doña María Apaza is not just any old lady, but I chose to introduce her without her titles because it's important to remember that she is also a human being like you and me. But now, let me tell you more. Doña María Apaza is the last high priestess in her lineage of the Incan Q'ero tribe in Peru, and she comes from a place in the world that has only been connected with Western culture for the past thirty years. Within the last year, she heard a call to action from spirit, and left the location of her Indigenous tribe in order to deliver her message of the heart. This means that she was sixty-eight when she learned news of the West and now at ninety-eight, she had been inspired to travel North America, on planes, to spread the gifts of her message.

Doña María Apaza arrived in a red long-sleeve shirt, a brown hat and a skirt, and sat like someone who had stayed close to the earth all her life. Evidently, through the way that she felt to me, she has nurtured that friendship. She was introduced as an Alto Misayoc whose title means, "She who welcomes the major spirits of the most important and powerful," and also that she had been hit by lightning twice. She shone bright like a star in the humble body of someone totally unassuming. As she spoke, we all listened, awaiting the double translation from her native dialect into Spanish and then into English. The intonation she brought forth danced, and the translation was an immediate reflection of the rippling affect her words had on those before her. Deeper than what was revealed on the surface, I could tell that this was a serious mission for her soul. Big Mamma was in the house. She was my answer key, and even though Doña María didn't speak to Alzheimer's, she showed me what it was like to live a lifestyle that had allowed her to remain healthy and thriving at ninety-eight, all while humbly honoring the earthly cycles of human life.

So, here we were. I was sitting in a chair beside my dear friend Megs as part of a small audience, listening to Doña María share her story as I quietly wept. Tears were swelling from my eyes, which were coming up from a deep place in my heart. Her presence had plucked a string within me tuned to the tone of truth. With a single pluck, all which was not vibrating in purity was wanting to be cleared away in the wake of its song. You could say it was a moment of resolution. Doña María asked us to come up to her in groups of four that day to receive a flower blessing, and as we did, these were the words she spoke (once they were twice translated), "Now that we've all been blessed with a sweet heart, may we live in harmony together. May we become one heart, and walk together on one path . . . until we don't. Thank you, brothers and sisters of my heart. Come back. Come back. May the spirit return."

As she spoke, I could feel a sense of light descending into the space, meeting each one of us as intimately as we would allow it. And I, a fountain of tears, was allowing it in pretty deep. My pearl at the bottom of the ocean was presenting itself, and it came in the form of a blessing through the sound of Doña María's voice. The full answer, not just in the words, but in the essence of those words and the vibration of the intention behind them. You see, the essence of the words embodied by the spirit of Doña María came from the Divine Mother and in alignment with her truest nature, she showed me that illness no longer served a purpose. Doña María was in balance with life, and inside her world there was no need for dis-ease to manifest.

Then, because of synchronicity (what happens when we are aligned with the flow of our own life force), I transferred the flower blessing that Doña María had shared into a palm-sized rhodochrosite crystal heart. A crystal, which arrived magically into my life only moments prior, and which has a story all its own to tell. But more on that later. Upon doing so, and with a sense of grateful receptivity, I no longer felt such a strong resounding oh shit in my mind. Instead, having found my pearl, I swam up to the ocean's surface and was now acclimating back toward the sun.

Chapter Two: Meeting Ms. J

When I was four years old, I can remember getting into the car with my dad and having him turn on the radio. There was a song playing and as much as any four-year-old could, I had a moment of revelation. "Dad," I said, "Why are most of the songs on the radio about love?" He looked at me and replied, "Well . . ." pausing to think, "love is really important to people." And then there was silence. I knew that I was tapping into something important, and yet that knowing was fading. There I was, four-year-old me, already beginning to forget the foundation of human essence.

***

Now let's fast-forward some twenty-five years. I want to take you to the first moment that I met Ms. J. She is the woman behind the inspiration for this book and our meeting happened one cold, but bright and sunny day in the middle of January when I walked into a new environment for the first time. I was enrolled in a program that trained people to become energy healers, and as a part of that program we attended clinics to put methods into practice. These clinics were located in spaces where the energy fields of our clients were going to be less powerful than our own. That's because no matter how much we understood from our textbooks, if our fields were not stronger than those of our clients, our clients would be affecting us more than we would be affecting them. As students, we were still developing our holistic power, so clinics were placed in areas where we could be of assistance. Places like centers for addiction recovery, eating disorder clinics, and my personal favorite, senior centers.

Let's say each human being is like a battery, and that sometimes we need a back-up battery to give ourselves enough power to make the more significant changes in our lives. Energy healers are the world's back-up batteries in the most literal sense. We are the humans who have trained in the art of directing universal energy through the human vessel for the charge of other people's batteries. Universal energy is unlimited, but we still need to have a strong voltage capacity, and this is something that develops through practice. We also have in-depth training in the universal truth that "true change first happens from within." We are a cohort of humans who understand the science of human programming through the intelligence of the human energy field.

The human energy field is the canvas of this healing profession, and it's more commonly known as the aura. It's the bubble of energy that surrounds and interpenetrates our body. I like to reference the *Vitruvian Man* drawing by da Vinci, or its introduction through the character of Phoebe in the TV show *Friends*. However, energy healing is more scientific than Phoebe's character would lead you to believe. Our aura has layers of structure and layers of fluidity, and these layers contain the data that connect us to the emotional, mental, spiritual, and physical aspects of who we are.

Then there are the chakras. They are spinning vortexes of energy that connect into the glands in our body, and are responsible for inputting and outputting all the non-physical vibrations we receive while we are experiencing life. All the noise, smell, chatter, light, everything direct and indirect, conscious and unconscious, subconscious and subliminal, gets inputted through the chakras. Actually, life experience gets imputed everywhere on our bodies as we breathe, but the chakras are the epicenters. Each chakra's vibrational intake is different, and corresponds to an aspect of our psychology and physiology, and to a particular bandwidth of color. In the world of energy, humans are considered to be a rainbow bridge of light, our souls the stewards of the planet, and our subconscious a memory keeper for mother earth. Humans are connected to the divine by birthright, something which fell away from our global teachings over time.

I met Ms. J on this day because the clinic I signed up for was located in a senior center. It was mid-day, and the room was peaceful and bright. Angelic vibes were abounding as the sound of the birds and the way the picturesque window framed the treed garden terrace created a soothing space cocooned from the bustle of society. It was an ideal place to step in for healing; the space emanated serenity. I partnered up with a fellow clinician, and we were informed to expect a client who was experiencing Alzheimer's who had recently broken her hip. It was Ms. J. She came in guided by her daughter and sat down in a chair to receive her one-hour treatment. With a tuft of her silver hair flickering, she smiled and said, "Thank you." I lovingly attuned to her the way that I do, and as I did, I quickly gained awareness that something was not quite the norm. I had heard of Alzheimer's disease, but I had never come into contact with someone experiencing it. I missed taking in its weight when my teacher informed me of Ms. J's condition. There I was, spirit ablaze, training in the trenches of life, and I quickly realized that my tried and tested script was not going to cut it this time.

If you've never received an energy healing treatment before, allow me to explain the process. A typical client will lay clothed and face up on a massage table. It is a precious hour to themselves, and a repose from the busy world. They close their eyes, and within a matter of moments, surrender into a receptive state of rest. Energy healing consciously directs harmonious and resonant frequencies into their biofield, and this can make them feel sleepy. Your first energy healing session is often a lovely energetic massage for the mind, body, and spirit.

However, Ms. J was not my usual type of client. She was experiencing the advanced stages of cognitive decline of a dementia condition that was likely Alzheimer's disease, and there were a couple of other differences too. The first, was that she was sitting in a chair instead of laying on the table because of her hip injury. She nervously looked around the room as she rhythmically tugged at the hem of her sweater, and in the most innocent and naive way, she would ask in repetition, "When will this be over?" Despite all the awkwardness and nerves that were bubbling up from inside me, I attempted in earnest to acclimate to someone who was no longer fully present in this realm.

The second and more intriguing difference, once we made it through our introductions, was how easy it was for me to love her. There was a level of easefulness, which surprised me and that I've often reflected on. I imagine that for the caregivers who are reading this, those in the trenches and experiencing the decline of a loved one, there is a realization that you must be present for the moments you have left together. But easy love would not be the first words that come to mind. So, let me explain. When I am with a client, my heart-centered nature is one of my biggest tools, and it is also my gift. I can sense how my clients are feeling on the inside, sometimes even more than they can themselves. With Ms. J, the feeling of love I'm talking about is the one that comes from the presence of unconditional love. It's a connection inside oneself to a tangible state of self-acceptance and with Ms. J, despite all the awkwardness happening on the outside, on the inside there was this undeniable easefulness (one that most humans with a well-functioning mind don't commonly possess), and it was so curious to me.

As any good detective would, I've given myself time to investigate and do research on this moment, and I've decided that the ease I experienced with Ms. J was caused by these major influences. The first influence was Ms. J's relationship to her daughter. A relationship of true devotion and care, and one that fostered a sense of safety. Ms. J felt safe as her sense of self changed daily, and I was grateful for this because it was also this dynamic that set the stage for Ms. J to feel safe with me. The second was the effect of the threads of life tapestry aligning perfectly in more than one dimension. In other words, the second influence was mystical, and it included a connection between our souls. The third influence was how the rigidity of the mind, in its absence, was ceasing to limit the vastness of Ms. J's beautiful heart. This first meeting with Ms. J was a meeting that would change my life. I had no idea that an entire year would pass before I would meet her again, and that she would become one of my most interesting case study clients. Today, I only knew today, and I did not anticipate in any way what was about to happen next.

Full disclosure, my relationship with Ms. J started out rocky. Societal norms expect us to act in certain ways, but when someone is experiencing Alzheimer's, most of those norms are tossed out the window. During the initial moments of my experience, I was self-conscious. I thought, *If only she could grasp that this room was meant to be a silent one!* One part of me embraced her innocent banter, while another part desperately wanted to place her back into the structured box of our society. Unfortunately, controlling others was not a superpower I possessed. Humans aren't designed to control others anyway, and attempting to do so creates a lot of wasted energy. It never ends well either. If we have enough awareness to catch ourselves in the act of wanting to control another, what we can do is aim to redirect our efforts toward responding to our own impulses with compassion and understanding. It's from a place of quietude, once we find it, that we can then lovingly guide others, and even then, the truest form of guidance always comes from within.

My mind was spinning and my shoulders began to slouch. Control is based on attachment, and sometimes those attachments are deeper than what is conscious for us, which means they are impulses attached deeper than what we can easily change, and so stopping the pain is temporarily beyond our reach. I was having trouble holding space for all of Ms. J's box-breaking actions, but this time my attachment to the outcome didn't last long because in the next instant my healer heart kicked in. I spontaneously had the urge to expand more of my presence into the moment and to be unflinching with what was. I continued to breathe through my heart and as my breath expanded, something shifted. As I breathed in presence and acceptance, the colors in the room became more vivid, and without either of us moving a physical inch, I felt Ms. J move closer to me. She became the only other person in the room. The buzz in my mind faded, and I found myself resting there deeply in the heart space, with my newfound and vast level of compassion. My judgment left, and when she spoke I accepted what came through as right and normal. I was tuning into her version of reality. That is the power of an open heart.

In moments, I held her hand or gently placed my hand on her arm so that she could feel that someone was there with her in this new environment. My heart center continued to open until it felt like it was a flower in full bloom facing into the sun; a heavenly sensation. Ms. J and I rested there together for some moments and then two short sentences came through her lips; the first sparks of ignition for what was to become *Sparks from the Heart*. Ms. J turned to me and said with some confusion, "Oh . . . so did you just go and come back? You were just there, and now you are here." I sat with her question for a split second, and much to the skepticism of my rational mind, which greatly disliked the feeling of not being in charge, I responded to her query with, "Well, I'm a **channel**, so I can be in both places at once." I remember being shocked at what I had said, but this moment was only the tip of the iceberg to a much longer process of gathering and deciphering information. In that moment I was shown a door into another place, invited as a witness to Ms. J's sense of awareness as it moved from one reference point of experience into another. We met in a place where worlds seemed to overlap, and long enough for her to point at the clinic door (where there was no one), and say as her face melted with love, "Hey, there's my good friend over there." I nodded and smiled, and couldn't help but wonder if her good friend had already passed away. That Ms. J was meeting her in a place somewhere in the beyond. A meeting of souls to which I was also privy.

***

During my time on earth, training to be a healer has led me to believe that unconditional love is a birthright that comes with being human. It is a quality inherent in the heart and when we are in the presence of it, it feels easy, safe, and soft. Maybe you have someone in your life that makes you feel this? Perhaps a wise grandmother, who when you were young you could tell anything to, or a mentor you met along the way who softened into your trials and tribulations of life to lead you in the right direction. This is the love I'm talking about. It is the quality of allowing what is to exist without judgment, and it is the first step to any personal transformation. For most of us, we have to practice the art of acceptance for unconditional love to become our dominant program. At this time on our planet, in an age of powerful minds, unconditional love requires cultivation.

Chapter Three:
The Soul-Self Human Template

Perhaps, like you, I didn't grow up in the metaphysical world. I experienced a spiritual awakening when I was twenty-four, and I met Ms. J when I was thirty. Before these events, I was an atheist, and before that, I was raised Catholic. My journey has been an ever-expanding process of experiencing, believing, and then doing the research, in order for my sense of self to embody the vaster truths that became available to me. At twenty-four, I discovered the power of my heart, and I learned that I have the tendency to live strongly through it. This tendency makes me an empath, and mystical experiences are something I feel and receive through **claircognizance.**

Since my awakening, I've done a lot of living in the world of the healing arts, and I've noticed that the way we categorize mystical experiences is also expanding. Mysticism is not exclusively for esoteric people because it can be translated into an awareness of our subtle sense perception and this is a capacity that is inherent to all of us. It only needs activation and cultivation to blossom, and excitingly it's a part of our evolutionary progress. It's humanity's birthright to perceive beyond the physical world, so I think it might be interesting for you to hear some of my day-to-day examples. This way, you may become aware of these subtle sense perceptions for yourself (if that's something that you'd like to do).

1) I walk into a party and there is a woman who feels nice to stand beside. Since her presence feels good to me, I choose to stand beside her and naturally, we start chatting. Later on, she tells me that we have a mutual friend who has spoken kindly of me in past conversation. In this situation, the first piece of information I received was felt—I could feel her anticipation and good intentions emanating towards me because of her open heart. Typically, in this type of situation, I'll find out the details of the story behind those feelings later on. I've learned that not everything has to be spoken in words to be known. It has also taken practice to discern if what I am feeling is about me or if it isn't—the feelings are not always good feelings, and it doesn't just happen with people. They could be feelings that come with places, nature, or maybe a certain book. In the world of feeling, messages pertain to the essence of things; the tone of a conversation or what's infused into an inanimate object.

2) I once spent an unexpected three hours meditating and cleaning out my jewelry box after a women's retreat. What started as a simple impulse to clean, evolved into a meaningful shamanic journey that wove me through my past. As I held each piece of jewelry in my hand, psychic imprints and memories were shared. Gifts held good wishes from friends, while my favorites held the stories they had accumulated over the time they'd been worn. Never underestimate the power of your jewelry box to help you remember who you are and where you have been. All you need to do is hold your items in your hands and ask to feel their vibration through your heart. Breathe, and let it sink in.

3) I'm going for a stroll in the forest. I enter the state of simplicity that comes from just being. Nice, right? While

I am walking, I feel a flash of joy, and then I hear a faint breath in the air say, "Oh hello, so nice to meet you!" The whisper came from the left of me. Next, I might feel an overwhelming need to sit by a flower that also happens to be to the left of me and take the time to smell it. Nature does speak to us, and all of us have the capacity to hear her if we only choose to listen.

Not only did my experience with Ms. J become possible through my subtle sense perception (a topic that we'll continue to explore as this book continues), I also needed to have a conceptual understanding of what soul consciousness was. I needed to have a reference point for reincarnation, and life as the soul sees it after the one we are living is complete. In my experience with Ms. J, soul awareness became a part of our story, but it was also a part of my personal story long before we met. That's because after my awakening, I began to remember some of my past lives, and then sought out a world view that could explain my experiences to me. If you are someone who has never considered the topics of soul or past lives before, try and keep an open mind, and if you are someone who is finding that to be difficult, that's okay too. Your questioning is welcome. In fact, it's a sign of intelligence.

The essence of your soul (a concept that we'll also continue to explore as this book continues), is the part of you that is cultivated through long-term experience, and by long term I mean thousands of lifetimes long. We also live lives between lives[1] and if you are someone experiencing Alzheimer's in your life, investigating this topic can help you to better understand where your loved one has gone. Investigating the concept of past lives is also a fun way to learn about yourself, as they can bring insight into why you hold a particular perspective, emotional tendency,

---

1   Michael Newton, *Journey of Souls: Case Studies of Life between Lives*. Woodbury: Llewellyn, 2000.

talent, pitfall, or gift today. They are underlays to your current life, and they offer you a more profound understanding into your soul's background. Consider them like a curriculum vitae through less narrow eyes.

Relating to the concept of soul, we arrive at your first framework, which I've called the Soul-Self Human Template. The ideas it explores are intended to create room for expanded contemplation on how illness gets created by offering you a more expanded concept of who you are. As a soul, each lifetime that you live is an evolution from the previous one, and although your remembrance of those many lives is wiped from your awareness, so that you can impactfully immerse yourself in the moment, your soul will still carry that evolution forward through your essence (which is something you can sense into in this lifetime). The pinpoint expression of who you are now can also be expanded to embrace more of this essence, and that is the purpose of this template. Through the lens of illness, it's a template that can help you to see in a less personal way (perhaps in a less self-critical, and less fear-based way too). While from a space of self-discovery, it's a template that can help you to become more aware of your broader uniqueness as an individual. There is a deeper reason for why we all look, see, think, and feel so differently, and we can explore it because it's coded into our souls.

The Soul–Self Human Template

1) *Your Family Lineage:* All the pains and losses, as well as the joys and accomplishments from your family lines, are programmed into your DNA. You become a unique fusion of your father's family line, and your mother's family line. You inherit their beliefs, their emotional responses, their inclinations, their physical features, their history, etc. All of this becomes a part of who you are.

This is biological, yet it can also be transferred through time spent, especially your emotional responses, beliefs, and inclinations.

2) *Your Soul History:* Every incarnation you've ever had (not all of them necessarily human) yield experience and wisdom, and these experiences mix to become your essence. Like your family lines, these experiences can include wounds and gifts. Oftentimes, we will incarnate into a family that will reflect or vibrate similarly as our soul heritage. In a broader sense, you already were that which you incarnated into. Yet, nuances definitely exist, and it does help to have two categories.

3) *The Location of Your Incarnation in Time and Space:* When you are born, the outside world offers you new experiences to create the most updated version of who you are. This includes your city (or birth location), your country, your school, your family dynamic, your neighbors, the media, television, music, school, and more. Experiences from the outside world are especially influential until the age of seven, as your chakras don't yet have filters on them. Everything that you experience up until this age goes directly into the quantum aspect of your cells, becoming the baseline program for the rest of your life.

4) *The Alignment of the Cosmos During Your Birth:* The energy of the planets and their constellations as they were at the time and date of your incarnation inform the qualities and tendencies that create the template for your character and life path. Your personality and the uniqueness of your healthy ego, is a cosmic template, which has been gifted to you from the planets and stars. (I've always found it fascinating how it's the billionaires and the free spirits that seem to take the science of astrology most to heart).

Lastly, add in the **soul contracts**, which you signed before you were born, and you'll get a pretty expansive overview of who you are and why you are here now. All of these factors are what create our first template. This template will be our launching pad, so take a couple of breaths and check in with yourself. Take notice if this is the type of perspective that you'd like to keep exploring.

***

When I realized that I would be turning my thoughts on Alzheimer's into a book, I knew that I would need more experience with those who were living with the disease. So, I volunteered at a day program for people experiencing dementia, and that's where I met Mr. M, a former hockey coach. He wore a big gold ring as proof, but that's as much as I knew about his past. Mr. M didn't say much anymore, and when he did, it was usually something like, "Well, what are you going to do with that?" or, "I'm just going to go." Luckily, there were many loving and kind souls volunteering at the day program, that when he did feel the need to get up and go, he was kindly guided back into the group, or they'd find him an activity that he liked to do, such as helping with the required daily tasks.

The lunchroom at the day program was cozy, and the staff adorned the tables with bright-green and blue tablecloths, and vases of flowers. It had community center vibes, and as much as it was a space created for people experiencing dementia, it could have just as easily been a space for a knitting club or a committee meeting. The space emanated connection. For lunch, we sat, ate, and socialized. There were four or five people to a table and sometimes, along with lunch, there were games. On this particular day, a *What Would You Choose* card was placed in the center of the table (a card to probe a question). During my time as a volunteer, these types of conversations quickly became my favorite way to pass the time. This crew was not afraid to speak their truth. It was the perfect combination of symptoms mixed with age; joie de vivre graced this room and I thoroughly enjoyed the freedom in their state of mind. It was a space cultivated through safety, simple structure, and an open heart.

Today, the question for the table was, "What would you choose: to live two hundred years in the past or two hundred years in the future?" All four of us ladies had a quick reply. It was a no-brainer, the 1820s, and our reasoning . . . the fashion! Then it was Mr. M's turn. He sat there, pondered for a moment, and then decided that he'd choose the future. "Ah! So, you want to go to outer space?" responded one volunteer. "Well, why not," smirked Mr. M with a laugh, "I spend most of my time there anyway!" We all giggled, and I could sense the honesty in his response. I don't know for certain where the **astral plane** is located physically in time and space (perhaps it's located outside these), or the location of where the soul goes after we die, but I could feel some truth in his retelling. Just like Ms. J, most of Mr. M's consciousness was no longer located on earth in the here and now.

In the game *What Would You Choose*, Mr. M chose the future, but let's take a moment to go back into the past. That's because I'd like to take you back to my time spent with Ms. J; a year after our first session, I met her again as my case study client. We did a series of eleven treatments together once a week and I learned many things. Then, as I was writing my final paper some months after that, there was a moment when I could sense her spirit nearby. After a day of hitting walls in my research paper, I was driving home, crying, and questioning *(alone in a car can be a great place for emotional freedom)*. Immediately, a wave of psychic story came through that brought me to even more tears, and I felt the purity of my curiosity and good intentions acknowledged by Ms. J's spirit. She was making her support clear. Ms. J's daughter had told me that from the age of eighteen Ms. J had been a school teacher, and that she loved her job. I remembered this and felt highly attuned to her passion to guide and share knowledge. It confirmed for me that Ms. J was still connected to the happenings here on earth, and because her consciousness was across the veil, that she could also see things differently.

***

It is the natural course of life to be born and then to die. This has been going on for eons. What's unnatural is that we don't talk about death enough. It's also unnatural that when Al is present, the soul of that person can leave this dimension, while still remaining connected to their human body. In the traditional death process the soul leaves fully, arrives in a space of life between lives, and the body is no longer animated, but in Alzheimer's the soul seems to be confused about its permanent address. "Why?" I wondered, and after two years of detective work on the subject, my thoughts arrived at this: no matter if we are here embodied in our incarnation, or if we are hovering somewhere ever close to our earth-life on the other side watching in, from a space of higher knowing, both experiences are equally a part of God. Although Alzheimer's disease is pulses away from our birthright to be healthy, the experience is still of benefit to the soul because to a soul in this world everything is a balancing act. Alzheimer's may be a way to balance a more extreme imbalance, but its outcome is balanced nonetheless. There is a reason that the soul has chosen to fracture its experience in this way, and perhaps the answer is unique to each family that this choice affects. My heart also tells me that if we find ourselves still here on earth, in whatever shape or form that may be, we are here because we still have a mission to complete.

Chapter Four:
Walking the Worlds

I'm curious, how are you doing with all this metaphysical talk of souls, the astral plane, and reincarnation? I suppose if you are still with me, you're finding it interesting. It took me a process of eight years to get to the place that I am today, so I wonder what effect this vantage point has on someone who is entirely new to this version of reality. Spiritual awareness is about attuning yourself to the subtle nature of things, and it takes time for the body to evolve into being able to hold a more conscious awareness of those subtleties. But like I said in the previous chapter, it is a capacity inherent in everyone. It's just a matter of where you choose to place your focus, and how much you choose to practice.

We won't be speaking about the most well-known version of Al, as he shows up in the later stages of human life (much further in the book), but I do promise we'll come back to him. Instead, we are going to switch gears for more preparation, and before we get into more of your training, I think it would be wise to share my journey as I've travelled it. This way, you get to know a little more about the messenger behind the message, which tends to make the message more meaningful.

I grew up the eldest of three girls and as far as normal goes, I fit perfectly into that category. I never noticed that

I could or should be aware of more in my reality, except for one or two little things here and there. As a child in Catholic school, the most endearing memory I have of my relationship to my soul was in my first year of kindergarten. It happened while sitting in a morning circle, when we were taught the *Hail Mary* prayer—which I already knew by heart. I recited its words with familiarity, and I went home that afternoon knowing that I was *totally kicking it* with Mother Mary. As a child, I was shy and sensitive, so instead of telling my parents, I deduced that what I felt was definitely impossible because Mary was a famous lady written about in the Bible. Still, something in my heart told me she lived in me too. She felt like immense unconditional love, I just didn't have the right worldview to understand it yet.

Other than feeling that I knew Mary personally, and asking about the song on the radio while I was driving with my father, if I had to choose a spot in time when my interest in the meaning of life began, I would turn back the clock to the summer between grade ten and eleven. That summer, my friend Penelope and I travelled to the Island of Crete, while our journey to get there began the previous winter. We were hanging out in the guidance office of our high school when something caught our eyes. There on the little rack that dressed the waiting area was a brochure advertisement for summer school abroad in Greece. Not just any summer school either, it was uniquely to study grade eleven English. The class that was notoriously known in our high school to be the most difficult and the most workload-dense of any other. The opportunity we had discovered seemed to us like finding buried treasure—and it was. Crete opened me up to contemplation and invited me on a lifelong journey into the wisdom of living.

There we were, my first time on a plane and my first time abroad. Crete was an adventure. We had all new classmates, a built environment that suddenly became white terraces and terracotta set against the epic blues of the ocean, and a deep and wise philosophical mind for our teacher. A philosophical mind that had us read a book called *Blindness* by Jose Saramago and write in daily journals as part of our course work. Journals which he would sometimes read aloud to the class. I seemed to have forgotten the out loud part one day as I wrote a particularly angry entry cursing my beloved travel companion. Through the lens of my teenage mind, Penelope was getting on my nerves, and it was of course that day of all days that our teacher chose to read my journal to the class. Chaos ensued, and I learned in a convoluted way (whether they are shared aloud by an eccentric teacher or not), that no secrets are truly secret. Eventually, everything will come into the light. It was a good first introduction to the power of presence and energetic principle. I now understand that when we hold on to secrets, less of our truth can express itself in the present. We think that we are hiding pieces of ourselves from others, but we are firstly hiding those pieces from ourselves, and that locks energy in the past that would otherwise be accessible to us in the now.

We took a bus to school every day, down a winding, bumpy road on the edge of a mountain. A journey that was decorated with white crosses honoring those who died driving too fast or in bad weather, and they were humbling to me at a young age. One month in Crete and I was effectively faced with contemplating death. The road was also lined with funny-looking buildings. They looked part home with traditional doors, windows, and walls native to the land, and part parking garage, with concrete and rebar shooting up from the second or third story pillars holding everything together. They overtly portrayed themselves as being unfinished and when I questioned my teacher, he explained to me this: mortgages in Crete were not commonplace, so people would build what they could afford and leave the rest for later. Then as time went by, and their family grew, they could add new floors with relative ease. This was another moment of revelation for me. Their approach to building seemed full of multi-generational love, and I decided then and there that I wanted to become an architect.

Seven years later, I was in my second year of architecture school, but also in a lot of pain. "It's the darkest before the dawn" is what they say, and my darkest hours were probably at this time in my life. I remember it feeling like all of my dysfunctional habits, which included addiction, codependency, and emotional repression, spilled over and out into the world with the breaking of my heart. It was not something I expected (nobody plans a breakdown), since the year before had been the most amazing dream. I had been accepted into the architectural design program, was excelling in something that I loved, and to top it all off I had fallen in love. *Sigh.* I remember the first time I said *I love you* vividly. The early morning sun was glistening onto the wall where we sat reading side by side, and I just felt like saying it. "I love you." Those three simple words that can change everything. Three years my senior and someone I adored, he looked at me, smiled, and then he said it back. I sensed a bubble form around the two of us, and for a time, it was bliss. It's in those moments when you least expect it that love finds you, and for the first time ever I felt I was living life with both feet in the water.

While living in this love bubble, there was an area outside the architecture building where we used to drink coffee and smoke cigarettes, and just to the left of that space was a basement level rock garden. It was a rectangular space carved out of the earth, which you would get to by a set of concrete stairs. The architecture building where I attended school was built in 1968 in the architectural style of brutalism, and although purposeful intention brought with it a particular charm, the surrounding spaces were also heavy and bleak.

On this particular day in the rock garden there was a group of us smoking, and for me, it was the first time in a day-lit setting that I chose to smoke cannabis. I felt like I was crossing a line, and I chose to cross it because of curiosity and because of peer pressure. Soon afterwards, and high as a kite, I then decided it was time to go home. Something unique happened in the moments while I sat waiting for the bus. A sensation arose within me, in the shape of a ball that felt like a spinning vortex inside my chest. Something that I had never felt before and something I assumed was just a part of the experience that smoking created. Yet, when I followed up with my friends the next day, they listened, stark faced and aloof. It wasn't until years later in the energy healing program that I attended, that I learned I was feeling one of my chakras.

Getting from point A, the one smoking outside the school basement, to B, the one who was attending what would be best described as a very unassuming and very Canadian branch of Hogwarts School of Witchcraft and Wizardry, was actually a treacherous journey. Substance abuse and mild addiction, like a handshake from the dark side of solace, first came through to greet the emotional pain that I didn't even know I had. Over the course of my short-lived relationship I had started to dress like my partner, I cut my hair short like his, and I began to like what he liked: MDMA, nightclubs, and nightly alcohol became a part of my reality. I lost myself. The thing is, you don't know that you are losing yourself until it's too late. It's only when that person you lost yourself to is gone that you begin to notice. When we broke up only eight months after that fateful day in the sunshine, I was numbed out, having trouble staying focused, and aimlessly looking for my other half. I had never felt so much pain.

Then one day, months after we had broken up, in that same place where we used to smoke cigarettes and drink coffee, I held in my hand a list of study abroad options. It was perfect timing. I knew that I needed a breath of fresh air to move me through the darkness I was feeling, and this seemed like my ticket. For years, I held a dream that I would spend my exchange term in Paris. I had fallen in love with the city while working there as a nanny in years past, but this was an unexpected turning point. As I scanned the page before me, my pointer finger grazed the list: Berlin, London, Madrid, Paris, and it kept going . . . and then stopped like a magnet at Pune . . . INDIA. India. I took a breath and felt the flutter of a soft caress in my heart. And just like that, like a wave receding into the ocean, my old dream was washed away. A new pathway had appeared.

Chapter Five:
India and the
Wind of Change

India has some of the best and worst smelling scents I've ever smelt. In one walk down a city street, you might get a whiff of burning garbage on garbage day, then turn the corner to receive a 180-degree transformation and be greeted by the mouthwatering combination of crisp cilantro and cooking spice. And the colors, oh the colors! Saris in unlimited hues would light up my vision like rainbows every time I walked down the street, but that was just the beginning. No matter where I went, and during all the new experiences that life had in store for me, it seemed that whenever I stopped to pause, the old shadow would creep in. I was addicted to going back in time and to the way I felt when I first fell in love; the grasping and clinging were taking control. Despite the rationalization from my mind that it was an experience which had run its course, I was stuck because my heart was still healing.

Studying at an all-girls architecture school in India taught me two new lessons. The first is the goodness that comes from building in alignment with the earth. There was a joy that sprang up in me when I saw how this culture would build their patios and homes around the trees. They would adjust the built environment to fit into nature, allowing trees to block what would otherwise be a passageway or leaving them to grow into the building. I don't know the practical reason for their choices, but to my heart it felt respectful and wise. How many times have you gone for a walk in the forest, and how many times has it made you feel better than you were feeling before? The idea of bringing this experience into our daily life by including a tree in the home, inspired me to move back towards nature as well. In school, they taught us to align our buildings with the movement of the sun, how to incorporate organic airflow, and the importance of working with local and natural building materials. These practices became the premise for their designs, whereas in the West, during my education, they would have only been a consideration. In my time spent in India, I relished in a renewed sense of kinship with the natural world.

The second lesson was how to work together. Coming from a Canadian school where individual self-expression dominated our studio classes, working in a **co-creative** dynamic was a shock that required a lot of softening on my part. A softening that would take a lot longer than four months in India, but it was a start. One night, a group of classmates invited me over for dinner and homework. I was stunned as I watched them lay sprawled out on the floor, passing around papers and sharing answers. This was not what I was expecting. The prestige in me was appalled, yet my sense of belonging was ever so curious. I had no idea how to respond, but I could acknowledge that this was an experience that felt better than what I was used to. It pointed out to me that somewhere along the way, I had removed myself from letting in the simplicity of loving comradery.

There were three of us from my Canadian school who traveled to India and because I was experiencing heartache, I decided that I needed to live alone. Of course, at that time,

I had not yet connected the dots. Outside of school hours, I turned into an island, and reruns of *Sex and the City* became my new best friend. I smoked cigarettes from my third story window hidden in the trees, and I finally had the space to acknowledge how sad I was. I contemplated that drinking wine every night to soothe the voices was not the best way to deal with my emotions. But it was all that I knew.

In my early weeks in India, I began to hear the word "meditation" and it made me remember something that I had read in a book. The book was *Eat Pray Love;* a classic by Elizabeth Gilbert. Appealing to my wandering spirit, she wrote about her experience with meditation, and I recalled how she had created a sense in me that there was more to this life than meets the eye. As an architect in training, she made me feel deep in my bones that an empty white space might be the most profound. She'd struck a chord, and I knew that meditation had something to do with it. On any given week, the word would fly through casual conversations with other foreign exchange students and on an exceptional day in my personal history it was even paired with the word free. "I did a retreat once," my tall, dark-haired and handsome exchange student friend explained, "it was ten days in silence, and it was free. If you have the means, you can give a monetary donation, but what they really love is if you donate your time in future courses. They have them all over India, and it's called Vipassana."[1]

The options for meditation I knew thus far were luxurious retreat centers aimed at rejuvenation and relaxation for Westerners that also came with steep Western pricing, or boho hotspots to connect with others, do yoga, and party. Neither of these were what I was seeking, but this

1   Vipassana Meditation (website), accessed February 7, 2021, https://www.dhamma.org

new offering made me light up. Through my student budget-colored glasses, the word *free* grabbed my attention, and I wondered about this mythical place on earth where everyone who had the desire was allowed to learn to meditate. Meditation had grown into something that fascinated me. I knew in some way it would help me, but it also scared me. Not because I was afraid of what I might discover about myself (that was where the fascination came from), but because I was afraid of walking a new path and moving away from what I had known. Intrigued, I asked my friend to tell me more, and I listened with a flame ablaze in my eyes. I knew I was one step closer.

In Pune (pronounced Pu-Nay) the city of my four-month home, there is a well-known ashram, which is a place devoted to religious or spiritual pursuit. This particular ashram was founded by a man named Osho—a controversial and beloved spiritual leader who died in 1990. We traveled there as a class one afternoon to study the meditation pyramid, and I found myself secretly enchanted by the small bookstore by the entrance instead. It was there where I bought my first two spiritual books: *I Say Unto You* and *The Path of Meditation,* both by Osho. His words simplified the world in a way that I had never been exposed to before. I've realized over time that it's important to understand the simplicity in a subject before we can start to make things complex, and Osho made life less complex in a way that nourished my spirit. I read his books like I used to read *Harry Potter*, with intrigue and envelopment, and quickly. Everything he said was new information, and it stirred an old knowing of a truth deep within from a place I had not yet discovered.

I booked my Vipassana meditation retreat in Lucknow soon after. Well, I should correct that sentence—I emailed the retreat center and assumed I booked my Vipassana retreat in Lucknow soon after. Then, once the school months passed, I began some planned traveling before reaching my final destination. These travels included a stop in Bangalore and Pondicherry; Bangalore, to visit a cherished family friend, and Pondicherry because it was colonized by the French. I had an affinity to French culture, so to see French–Indian fusion from an architectural perspective was something that intrigued me. However, I was still learning to connect with the earth, and forgot about the importance of checking the weather. I don't recall much of my time spent in Pondicherry because of the heat, the sun was so hot that I could barely make it down the street. Yet, there was a silver lining because I could do something that I have never been able to do again, which was to practice Bikram hot yoga (traditionally held in 40-degrees Celsius heat and my favorite form of exercise), from the comfort of my very own hotel room.

Very close to Pondicherry, there is a place called Auroville, and it instantly attracted me. Acquaintances described a big meditation sphere in the center where all races were welcome. When you look up Auroville's website they say that, "Auroville wants to be a universal town where men and women of all countries can live in peace and progressive harmony, above all creeds, all politics, and all nationalities. The purpose of Auroville is to realize human unity."[2] I was at a crossroads between worlds, and when I read their intention through the mindset that I carried in university, it included visions of red flags coming straight from the cult-o-meter itself. But the part of me in the other world was stronger, and who I am now vouches for those words completely. Once you step onto the path of awakening, explanations like the one above become much less cultish and much more like embodied and known experiential truths. Words like these come from

2   Auroville (website), last updated November 18, 2014, www.auroville.org/

the deep truth of the human heart and the embodiment of a more expanded sense of awareness. No one is forcing you to adopt them either, on the contrary, to get to this place you are encouraged to question, contemplate, and claim your discoveries for your own. It's like walking through a portal into another density of reality while still being able to stay grounded in the things you've known from before. On the other side of the portal, things are softer, slower, and full of substance because people have learned the joy of living that comes through a balance between being and doing. It's a portal which is offered to everyone.

As it was with my visit to Auroville, the heart will *pull you* toward places that it resonates with most because the heart's subtle energy field is electromagnetic in nature. This magnetic pull happens before anything our five senses can interpret, as we just have that feeling or inner nudge at first. In the case of Auroville, once I started getting closer to it, my five senses did interpret the shift in frequency, and the air began to smell of sweet honey and freshly baked French bread. I remember it well. I remember being on my moped, taking in a big and grateful breath of goodness in that moment because it was such a stark contrast from the previous and more usual smell of garbage being cooked in the heat of the sun.

Now after you let out a gag or two, the lesson in this story is that goodness will give you clues when it's around, and on the journey of healing, your heart will lead you there if you listen. It goes without saying that the not so good will also give you clues into its essence because there are no secrets in the world of energy. I share my visit to Auroville with an intention to bridge the gap between the world that we live in and the one that is just around the bend. My time in Auroville was brief, yet impactful and in a synchronistic series of events to come, the teachings of its co-founder Sri Aurobindo, would later become the backbone of my training in the healing arts.

After Auroville, I travelled to my final destination, Lucknow, to begin my long awaited Vipassana training. When I arrived at the front reception a couple of hours late, I was greeted by an attendant who searched for my name on the list. I was not there. She then went to her superior, and he looked for my name on the list. It was true, my name was nowhere to be found. The superior began to ask me questions and as he did, he started to remember me. "Ah," he said, "yes, you emailed us, but we never responded to you. We didn't accept your application . . . but you are here now, so I suppose we can make some room." This was the moment that I started to question the power of my soul. Normally, I would have felt fear, or embarrassment, or I would have realized that I needed a confirmation email and not gone at all. But nothing seemed to phase me because there was a deeper and unwavering sense coming from within guiding me to where I needed to go. If the heart's pull is magnetic, I suppose it is the soul that keeps us centered in those moments of opportunity that will lead us back to our truest selves.

Inside the retreat, its attendants fell into unofficial yet distinct categories. Most were townsfolk, for them, it was a bit like a vacation that fit into their budget. They were served beautiful healthy meals, had time to themselves, and could practice meditating into the higher densities of reality. Then there were the nuns; they glowed, each with their head shaven and wearing different shades of orange. To watch them was like having a bright and sunny fall day stroll in and out of the meditation hall. Sometimes, while deep in their internal world, they would let out a very long and loud belch that erupted from deep down in their abdomen. It made me laugh and I was eternally intrigued. How were they getting so deep, and what was it they were clearing away? There was a thin influx of Westerners, a total of three including me, and halfway through for reasons unknown, we became only two. Finally, there was my saving grace—the well-to-do wife of a fabric store owner who could easily afford to pay for private quarters. When I showed up out of the blue, she offered that I may stay in her quarters with her and make use of the second bed. We slept in one small square room where each of us had our own bed frame, thin mattress, and a mosquito net. There was no talking. Every morning I would glance over as she would effortlessly fold and wrap her sari onto her body, and then lay it out flat to be folded again once it was no longer of use at the end of the night. In her fifties or sixties, with silver, shoulder-length hair, she was so beautiful to me. The details in the fabrics matched the detail she possessed in her self-care routine, and as a role model for the feminine essence, she was a gift to witness. At times these fabrics would be hung outside to dry and during one instance in particular, as I gazed out at the beautiful colors swaying in the breeze, the smell of incense licked my nose and the resident peacocks came strolling by to say hello. I felt like I was in heaven, and maybe I actually was.

Later on, I learned that there are Vipassana centers all over the world, and the ones I would attend in the future also had animal neighbors to remind me of this heaven on earth. In the silence and peace of meditation, I have seen a mother deer and her babies walk the sun-soaked trails through the long summer grass of West Coast America, not six feet from my own footsteps. While in the interior of the current province that I call home, I've played hide-and-seek with chipmunks. They followed me for much longer than a moment through the forest, hiding and seeking as I strolled. In what seemed to be propelled by the spirit of curiosity, the chipmunks' beating eyes would meet my gaze, and they were not the least bit spooked by my giggles.

Over the years I have taken part in five silent Vipassana retreats, each one very different, and dependent on what was going on in my life, but the first one was the most difficult. It wasn't until three years later, while in my fourth retreat, that a wellspring of compassion arose in me for the beauty and naive steadfastness that I portrayed in those early moments of learning meditation. How innocently I went marching into the fire without having any idea about anything. My twenty-something-year-old self sat in that room for ten days straight, bearing an excruciating level of pain. As my body adjusted to the aches that arose from sitting still, I dreaded the thought of creating movement, while I simultaneously broke that etiquette by turning my head to check the clock (every fifteen minutes). Plus, as some things were only said in Hindi, I missed all the cues for opportunities to meditate in the comfort of my room. As a warrior without any self-realization to the fact, I trudged through the pain and confusion, for some deeper reason that as a self-proclaimed atheist, I knew nothing about. I was a seeker before I knew I was seeking.

On day seven of my first retreat, I was meditating in a private cell; an opportunity which was offered to each of us a couple of times during our stay. I was meditating in a small room when I remembered a story the teacher Goenka had told us about a man who had created continental ballistic missiles with nuclear heads. Goenka explained that he'd walked by this man as he was meditating in his cell, only to find him standing on his shoulders as his whole body shook (as if he was possessed). It was his body's way of releasing the emotional and mental anguish he had created through his actions.[3] As I was alone in my own small cell, I thought . . . *what if that started*

---

3   S.N. Goenkaji, *10 Day Vipassana Course - Day 8 (English)*, YouTube Video. August 20, 2014, 62:57. https://www.youtube.com/watch?v=Us5Iq302eNU

to happen to me . . . apparently I felt I was just as guilty. Instead, something else quite unique happened. The air pressure in my ears began to change and a series of vividly lit images began to come into my mind in flashes. I travelled through a wormhole and into the light-filled cells of the beating heart of my first trimester self. Similar to how the flesh in your finger looks when you shine a flashlight through it, I was getting a firsthand glimpse into the inside of my mother's belly, and the instant I registered what I was looking at, it vanished. What remained was an overwhelming sense that it was time for me to go home. I felt the tug from my soul, and it was saying to me, "Hey sister, it's time to book it back to love land, enough of this self-hatred, enough with the unconscious self-harm. It's time to remember how beautiful you really are."

In the moments between my first awakening experience and leaving the retreat, I was torn. The teachings said that it would take lifetimes to reach enlightenment and so how could something so profound be happening to me—a mere university student looking for relief, and why had the process only taken seven days? Was it fake? It felt authentic. The rest of the retreat I walked around with an extra glow of angelic repose and wondered what it was that I had tapped into. While my rational mind spent time trying to put my experience into boxes, another part of me spent time leaning in. A new part of my consciousness was activating, and an ancient love was awakening from its slumber. What began to reveal itself at that moment has since become a continual unfolding of growth and expansion. And as it is unavoidable in this process, it has also included many contractions and the destruction of what no longer served my greatest goodness.

Chapter Six:
Tra La La,
Falling in Love

I went to my first meditation retreat intending to stop my depression and self-destructive habits, not intending to get a glimpse of an entirely new way of being that would ask me to change the course of my life. In my first month home from India I felt shocked, stunned, cocky, enveloped in a new zest for living, and I noticed a strong need to breathe better and more frequently. I felt different after returning home, but I had no context from which to explain it. In that first meditation retreat I discovered that there was a way to heal and that it didn't require self-medicating, searching for a diagnosis, or giving power away to medical professionals. As assistants to *team you* they can be of great service, we just need to remember who's in charge, and acknowledge the wisdom that comes through having a personal relationship with our own bodies. There was a reframing that was taking place, and it told me through small nudges and inner knowings that all answers came from within.

When you get a cut on your body, it heals. That's because it's innately human to be self-healing and this is in all aspects: mind, body, spirit, and emotions. The missing ingredient is that we need to take the time to slow down, self-reflect, and go within to turn up our personal power. The healing nature of our being can't keep up with the fast-paced reality of our Western society, and so our first task on this new journey is to take a step inward and bring our consciousness back into ourselves. We move it away from constant projection into the external world and with the breath, we place it back inside. This is meditation at a basic level. Even if we just meditate for five or ten minutes a day, it's a powerful shift from not doing it at all. To be with the breath, with ourselves, is a powerful force of self-healing and when I continued to practice meditation, there was a peace and tranquility that bubbled up from the depths, and I was hooked.

Then, in the months that followed, something again shifted inside me in a big way. It all began when I was sitting on the toilet in a stall at my local yoga studio. As I sat there and did my business, I became entranced by a poster taped to the stall door. Staring back at me in an ever so soft and loving way was a woman smiling. Her name was Snatam Kaur and the poster was advertising her tour as a musician. She wore white clothes and a turban, which I later learned came from the Sikh tradition. Her attire did make me feel different from her, yet my connection to her eyes and her smile outweighed my resistance, and I looked her up later that week.

Some friends and I had renovated our backyard garage into a studio, and that's where I was when I turned on her music for the first time. I was sitting at my computer designing, and as the music began, I felt the need to lie down on the couch and close my eyes. In a moment of wisdom, I listened to that inner nudge and surrendered into receiving the devotional and ever-loving melodies of the angelic voice that is Snatam

Kaur. I breathed in her music and then spontaneously, from a place deep within my heart, I started to cry. I wept and wept for something, for which my mind had no answer.

I would describe it as opening a door to one of your favorite places on earth, a place that had in the past been wiped from your memory, and as you have found it again, its remembrance becomes an overwhelming gift. The secret is that this most favorite place on earth is a place that comes from within you, and finding it again is sometimes a spontaneous act of grace. I was taken by my experience completely, and grateful to have had this moment of solitude from my housemates for its unfolding. That's because crying is vulnerable and from a scale of one to ten, one being a single tear and ten being uncontrollable weeping and wailing, I would have been an eleven. With my face scrunched up, tears welling from my eyes, and snot dripping from my nose, this was not my most attractive moment. After my wailing, I got up from the couch, cleaned my face, and looked out the window into our backyard.

Something was very different in the way I was perceiving. The trees were greener, the plants were more alive, and I could feel them with my inner knowing. They were no longer just images, or photographs separate from me. I now felt a true and real connection, like the way you would greet a dear friend, that came from a felt sense that permeated through my heart. I could feel mother nature smiling at me. "Dear one," she was saying as the trees swayed in the wind, and the birds chirped, and the garden grew, "I love you." Not only that, she was showing me the beauty that I was seeing and feeling before me was not separate from me. It was me. Mother nature was loving herself and saying in the most nurturing and unassuming way possible, like the archetypal eternal mother, "Come home child." In the week that followed, I fell in love with myself.

***

I have two awesome sisters, and the one in this particular story is fierce and kind; she's thirteen months younger than I, and knows me inside and out. During the time of this story, she was working as a bank teller and whilst in the throes of this new love affair I was having with myself, I jovially paid her a visit at work. I remember the moment well as I walked down the street in Ottawa where we lived, soaking in the sunshine and the street culture, vibin' high and walking with a bounce in my step. I was wearing a red dress patterned with tiny baby blue maple leaves and feeling like I had just won the lottery. I felt like a million bucks and paradoxically this valuable sense of internal love didn't cost me a thing. The joy I was feeling swelled up from the fact that I was a human being, alive, and breathing with a beating heart. I loved myself so much and didn't really know why. It was just a feeling that came forth from inside me. As the days passed and the feeling stayed, I questioned if I had a brain tumor or some drastic imbalance in my hormones that could have created such a change, but at this moment I was in love and enjoying the byproduct of some internal shift whose cause was unknown.

My sister had been my pillar for all the difficulties I was facing while grieving my first broken heart, and she was certainly not expecting such a jolly camper. So, when I got to my destination, she pulled me aside and asked in earnest, "Marnie, I'm just asking because I care . . . but are you on drugs? Why are you so happy . . . is everything okay?" I smiled and said, "I don't know . . . I'm just this high on life. Maybe this is what enlightenment feels like, or maybe it's the present moment. I don't really know, something is just different inside me." And I stayed smiling. My sister looked confused, but she trusted me and so her concern dissipated. She gave me a hug and I carried on my day strolling down the street in that new red summer dress that I loved so much, still feeling like a million bucks.

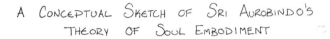

A CONCEPTUAL SKETCH OF SRI AUROBINDO'S
THEORY OF SOUL EMBODIMENT

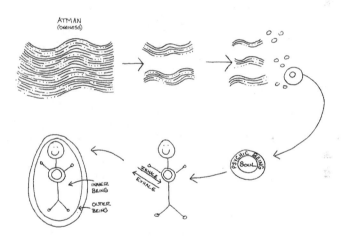

Many years later the yogic philosopher and twice Nobel Peace Prize nominee Sri Aurobindo, who created Auroville alongside Mirra Alfassa (another Divine Mother incarnate), put my experience into context for me. Sri Aurobindo held vast knowledge of what it meant to be human, and he wrote about it through a system which he called Integral Yoga.[1] It's a system that creates order, psychological thought, and poetic verse for the human experience, in a way which embraces the mystical and the mundane, and with a strong emphasis on the nature of the evolving soul. I studied his work over a period of five years during my training to become an energy healer—and I am still only grasping the tip of the iceberg as far as his brilliance is concerned. I have, however, learned enough to confidently share this, a portion of Sri Aurobindo's Integral Yoga Theory, which explains how the soul incarnates into our human vessels, or as I like to call them, our earth-suits.

I will begin the introduction to his theory by giving you a new word, and it's *atman*. In yoga, atman translates to essence or breath, and it is the substance that permeates all things. Atman, is another word for source consciousness or God, it's aliveness, it's oneness, and it's eternal love. Atman consciousness is bigger than our human cycle of life and death, but it also permeates our individual lives too because it is the essence of everything. Atman is the word that Sri Aurobindo uses to describe the fabric of life and as a self-reflective human being on this planet, it is our starting point.

Your second new word is *soul*. This word is common in our contemporary language, as most people have an idea of what the soul means. Plus, I've already offered you the Soul-Self Human Template, through which you can continue to expand and deepen that understanding. But, in the context of Sri Aurobindo's theory, the same word means something slightly different. For Sri Aurobindo, soul is the part of our essence that remains unchanged by experience. It is a small piece of the atman that has, like a river flowed

1   Ghose Sri Aurobindo, *A Greater Psychology: An Introduction to the Psychological Thought of Sri Aurobindo*, edited by A.S. Dalal. New York: Tarcher, 2002.

from the ocean, separated from its source to become its own stream of movement. It is perceived as separate from the atman, yet it is still made of the same fabric. It's like a river that trickles into a brook, that creates a pool, and that eventually becomes a single drop of water; it is separate, yet it is still the same.

To the human experience, the soul is the part of us that gives our bodies their animation. The human soul is like a drop of water, and it remains that drop of water through the construct of a human **ego** and physical body, while centrally emanating out from our subtle heart (anchoring also into the solar plexus and sacral chakra). Even though the soul is perceived as separate, from our vantage point here on earth, it still holds the possibilities contained in the fabric of the atman because it is one with it—just like a drop of water is a part of the ocean. It also means that the part of us that creates our aliveness has the same creative potential as God because it is a part of God. A big statement, which I interpret to mean that the soul, which incarnates through each of us, is responsible for creating our human reality in its entirety, both individually and collectively. We create our own earth-life reality (from inside the constructs of our human ego), and as we create and live, through the separate nature of the individuated soul, we remain individually and collectively the atman itself. In essence, it is a matrix illusion scenario.

On the soul level we are pristine everything-ness and beyond polarity; we are naive and all-knowing concurrently, and as a result, we are also void of the capacity to experience . . . because we are that which is beyond all experience. The soul is the unchangeable part of us, while this next concept is the part of our essence that builds up our soul-level curriculum vitae I introduced in chapter three, and our third term. Sri Aurobindo calls it the *psychic being*. If the purpose of being human is to learn and expand through experience, then the psychic being is the part of our energetic nature that grows outward from the soul as we evolve, to contain the memory of those experiences. The psychic being forms an energetic expression around the soul, which we create over lifetimes of living, and the continual inhale and exhale of our breath moves our experiences through the body, and directs them to be accumulated around the soul as it emanates out from the depths of the heart. I imagine it to be like an effervescent garden that continues to grow outwards around the elixir of life. It is our very own secret garden of wisdom, which becomes consciously accessible to us once we begin to look within.

Here at this deeper level within each of us, the psychic being is a mixture between our soul: an atman spark of eternal love, and the accumulation of our soul's experiences in its lifespan. Our inner gardens are effervescent and everlasting, and they may also be wildly amazing and out of control. This is because humanity, as a collective, has been living separated from its inner gardens for a long time, and although the essence of our garden is wisdom, not all of our experiences have been positive ones. The earth-life experience at present is a dualistic one, which means that the seeds of those experiences can be both negative and positive. If we haven't yet learned the lesson of a particular seed, that seed can still be growing strong and untamed. When we discover our inner garden, however, we have a new ability to become its caretakers and to weed out those seeds. We also have the ability to receive its amazing gifts; beautiful gifts which have grown forth from the elixir of eternal love itself.

There is uncharted terrain between the psychic being and the outward human experience in our collective history at this time, and this brings us to our fourth new term, which is *inner being*. This is the part of us that we begin to access when we choose to take our perception away from the outer world and sink into ourselves through activities like mindfulness, yoga, and meditation. The inner being is our inner world, and it's the place where we can become more familiar with our programming: a mixture between the seeds of our inner garden and the new experiences we have incarnated into. The inner being is a topic that we'll continue to explore in this book, as this is where so much of our suffering is created from. Remember how I told you that you hold the history of your family lineage and that everything you experience up until the age of seven becomes your baseline programming for this lifetime? This also doesn't have to stay that way. By becoming a witness to the thoughts, emotions, and physical sensations that make up our programming, we can also reclaim our capacity to transform them.

The inner being, like the psychic being, is uncharted territory for many people at this time, and this leads us to our last new term from Sri Aurobindo, which is *outer being*. We are all familiar with this version of the human experience because it is the part of the human being that lives consciously in the outside world. Before my first awakening, it seemed to me like that's all there was, but it's only a portion of our conscious potential. The majority of humanity functions from here, and it's not a mistake by any means, instead it's the whole reason that our soul incarnated into this reality in the first place—to gain new experiences. Yet, it is my understanding that things are also changing on planet earth, we are becoming a more conscious species, and because of it more people than ever before are waking up to the deeper parts of themselves.

After awakening, the journey continues still. As we keep inviting the presence of our soul and the wisdom of our psychic being into our external reality, our human consciousness, and our learning also continue to expand. If we are diligent in our efforts to clean house of the outdated programs and patterns we find on that journey (what's stored in our inner being), there will come a lifetime where there will be no separation between the density of the outer being and the life-affirming nature of the layers that exist in our inner world. It's a pivotal moment in the evolution of being human, and since I only know of it in a poetic way, I felt compelled to write you a short verse in order to best portray its beauty.

Like a millennia-long sunrise over a
mountain's peak,
the light of the divine comes to illuminate
our material form.
The light itself, in the same way it is at the
mercy of the mountain's intricacies,
grows to illuminate the nooks and crannies
of our personality and knowing,
that were formed in the wake of its
separation from itself.
Once fully illuminated, whether mountain,
man, or woman.
We are then able to see the true beauty of
what is now within the light.
We are a love affair between the spirit of
the divine and matter;
a story that writes itself over time with
each and every breath that we take.
One informs the other until finally, two
become one.

One of the funniest memories during this intense time of inner discovery was when I asked aloud to the universe, "What is happening to me!?" I was having a moment, and not minutes later and at the risk of sounding crazy, my laptop turned on a video—on its own—of a vibrational activation sequence from YouTube that told me I had "seeded this awakening point in my consciousness from a higher part of my being for this exact point in my timeline." I was feeling connected to my **higher self** at the time, so I just went with it. My inner dialogue probably went something like, *Okay . . . so some part of me that somehow really feels like they have been sent here on a mission from outer space, has set up a checkpoint to activate me here on earth to remember that I am actually some badass inter-dimensional and galactic soul. Okay, yeah, I'll just go with that.* But in all truth and with as much seriousness that a phrase like this one can garner from the general public, it was a feeling that came to me from a level of cellular knowing that said it was real, and I trusted.

As we open up to our own natural truth (which usually requires making changes to our foundations), our relationships may also change; new friends may appear seemingly out of the blue, old friends may become more distant, and the relationships that can stand the test of time may morph and evolve. In my experience of this, I fondly remember time spent in a newly formed friendship. We were huddled around a brunch table in passionate whispers, discussing why everyone else didn't remember that they were souls in a body. Why everyone wasn't in on the joke, and if in fact something had gone wrong in the universal plan. One of my biggest questions as I went through this process of remembering my multi-dimensionality was: why wasn't everyone around me waking up too? And, over the years, this has become my answer: it has something to do with the force of light and our level of growth as psychic beings. Think density. We all have the same soul essence; the deepest part of us is equal, but the earth is filled with psychic beings who are enrolled in kindergarten all the way up to their doctorate, and so their light quotients will be different. From the inside, we need to have enough light quotient to pull us inwards from the matrix, otherwise we'll stay locked into the external world and never consider going deeper. We need to have a psychic being, which is developed enough to have an influence on the material world.

Unless you grow up in some secret lineage of light that raises baby Buddhas or something along those lines, most of us will have been raised in a way that pulls our consciousness into the outer world (or outer being), rather than have our consciousness be lovingly guided towards our soul. Once our awareness is stabilized in the outside world, our experience will stay as such until our psychic being has developed enough light quotient to pull us back inside, once our awareness is stabilized in the outside world. Therefore, nothing has gone wrong in the universal plan as I had initially thought, and that's because there is purpose, growth, and learning in the way things have been. Separation has been a fruitful learning platform for humanity; for our psychic being to be of service in the way that our outer being requires, it needs to first grow through experience, and each and every breath that we take in our separateness is what grows that energy. So, just in case you are feeling like I was, and find yourself questioning where you've landed, rest comfortably knowing that it's not whether one way is better than the other, it's more about ushering in the process of evolution from one way and into the next (if that is what your soul is calling you to do).

In my experience listening to Snatam Kaur for the first time since I was a child, my psychic being broke through, and the purity of my inner nature was able to reveal itself in my waking life. I fell in love with myself because I literally *fell into* the part of myself that is connected to the love of the atman. When I felt my inner goodness for the first time and realized that it emanated from within, it inspired me to make changes in the ways that I acted and thought, and the desire was strong and unwavering. In that sense, changing felt natural and effortless—yet from the perspective of my outer being there was much effort put forth. I learned that there is no way around life and facing its challenges, but there is a deeper level of supportive essence that is available for everyone to tap into.

We are also living in exciting times. The earth is going through an evolutionary shift in consciousness, which lightens the density of her reality. It's a shift that naturally supports our outer beings to vibrate more closely with the finer and lighter vibrations of our souls, creating a dynamic for our psychic beings to pull us back inside more easily. We are in the beginning stages of a collective rebalancing toward a vibration that is more connected to our souls. What seems to be forecasted is a global awakening for this decade, a mainstream remembering. Perhaps consciousness will become trendy in a real embodied way, and if it doesn't happen spontaneously, we are in a day and age of our story here on earth where we can consciously cultivate it. We can choose to search for our own soul essence if we find that it's not breaking through from the inside out. With conscious effort through tools like meditation and contemplation on goodness (as just some examples), we can allow this soul essence part of us to have more power in our lives.

***

Take a breath . . . take another big breath and take notice of your surroundings. Now, see if you can feel your heart beating. Smile. Check in. How are you doing? Perhaps you've already put the dots together: that a dis-ease like Al also has a first program. There is a part of Alzheimer's that is data stored in our subconscious (or inner being), and when we relate to it through our living individuality, Al's expression becomes unique. To be able to understand Alzheimer's in the way that I'd like to present it in chapter seventeen, the next five chapters are going to continue to introduce you to more theory, templates, and practical applications. They'll be less heavy on the story telling, as they aim to support you in seeing who you are in a different way.

It was Einstein who said that nothing is solved from the same level it was created, and an awakening—if you'd like to have one—comes with a whole new bandwidth of information to learn. What I am going to share with you next, is at times interactive, and if you feel called to participate, all you have to do is keep an open mind and soften your breath as you read on. If you choose not to participate, know that you can still read on and learn something new through your mind, without opening up to the changes that could take place. Due to the way this magic works, all you have to do is make the right choice for you, and your boundaries will be respected. If you read it once through, and then decide you'd like to come back and participate, you can always do that too.

Chapter Seven: Vibrate the Frequency of Your Divine Inner Child

Many years later, and back in my final year of training to become a healer, I had a client who I will call Dee. Dee was a cancer survivor and warrior of the highest caliber. She was articulate, resilient, and determined. When I met her, she was illness-free, yet she came to me holding on to grief from the years that she had just spent in the battleground of her illnesses. She told me that she had faced all the big hits with a stoic bravery, and that she now felt it safe to feel the enormity of everything she had gone through. On the first day that I met Dee, I could sense that an awakening had sprung forth from the depths of her heart.

There is a technique called "embodying a strength,"[1] which was taught to me in my training, and its purpose is to cultivate an internal feeling that connects you to your sense of strength from within. Through guided prompts, the technique is to visualize a scene that holds a meaningful positive and strong feeling for you, and then to link the felt sense that you've cultivated with a location in your body. This creates an internal resource for well-being that

---

1   Robin Fried, *Awareness Dialogue: Embodying/Anchoring A Resource* (Vancouver: Langara College Continuing Studies, 2019).

you can return to in times when you're feeling off-center, anxious, in fear, or looping through an old story in your head. It's especially helpful to have some of these in your tool kit if you choose to weed out your inner garden, but find your foundations becoming temporarily unstable as you do.

Without any talk of the soul or the psychic being, when I guided Dee to where she felt strong in her body she responded with, "My heart, and the words that go with its sensation, are forgiveness and enduring love." "Okay," I said, "and how do you know that?" Dee replied, "My inner child . . . she is in the green grass and looking around. A hummingbird flies over to her head, and it's beautiful. I know that magic is real here as I sit and am present in the nature that is before me. I know and I love so purely. That's me!"

As Dee told me this, she was tearing up from that overwhelm of love that she was experiencing from connecting to the version of her soul-self within. She was overwhelmed by the feeling of the deep purity of who she was, and that is the power of the soul. No matter the difficulty that is happening to us on the outside in life, this feeling is the trump card. Its knowing offers solace, it's where judgment dissolves, and a place that has the power to encompass our suffering with compassion. Once it's activated, it changes our reference point for living.

Dee's initiation into the deeper part of her soul was spontaneous, just like my own, but it is also possible to activate this initiation. Bashar, a non-physical being who was channeled by a man named Darryl Anka said, "This is not philosophy! This is physics! Everything is energy and that's all there is to it. Match the frequency of the reality you want, and you cannot help but get that reality. It can be no other way. This is physics."[2] What Bashar said is a foundational truth (a truth supported by Einstein), which rests in the knowledge that we are all vibrations of consciousness, that the law of attraction is real, and that we can match a vibration because humans have the capacity to be self-aware, to self-reflect, and to self-correct. The *knowing* that Dee and I both felt spontaneously is also a frequency that can be matched, and that's exactly what we are now going to do. In the next portion of this chapter, I am going to guide you through a process to activate the same energetic code within yourself. If you'd like to participate in this activation, breathe gently and softly as you read. While if you've chosen not to participate, you can treat what you are reading like a story, ignoring other directives in the future.

What does it mean to match a frequency exactly? A frequency is a moving vibration of energy, and before vibration becomes condensed into physical matter, it is sound and light energy full of information. Frequencies change based on the information that creates them, and so we can match a frequency by aligning our thoughts, emotions, and subtle sensations to the frequency we wish to match.

Choosing the right thoughts, emotions, and subtle sensations to align with us is a bit like choosing the right keywords to type into your Google search bar; they'll need to be specific and accurate if you are going to find what you are looking for. The questions to ask then become: what code are we trying to activate? And, what are the keywords that will help us to search for that code? The answer is written in the title of this chapter, *The Divine Inner Child*. This is the archetypal signature for the purest part of the human soul, it is the purity and love

---

2   "'The Ides of March,' Channeling from Bashar by Darryl Anka," Facebook Post, March 13, 2014, https://www.facebook.com/notes/3681234245241821/

that you were when you first entered this world, and it's the code for the interface between the atman and your human nature. Innocent and powerful, the divine inner child is the eternal love of God as God first steps forward into each unique human being. Humans are closest to the goodness of God (if they haven't yet cultivated their mystical heart) immediately after birth, and in order for that purity and wholeness to stay permeating through their cells as adults, they need to have lived in a way that has honored them. But first we need to remember that we are that beautiful child.

The next part of this chapter is dedicated to searching for this version of yourself within, and you can begin to soften into this way of experiencing by first stepping into the space of the witness. A good way to start is by following your breath inside and to start to see yourself the way you would watch someone you love; watching both outside of yourself and inside simultaneously. Over time, your ability to go inside will soften and open up, and you'll feel like you have more space. Like anything, it just takes practice and the possibilities are vast. Some yogis can see and feel into their organs, and I've even met one who could *almost* levitate.

If you are just beginning this inner journey, your mind will need some training. For most of us, the mind has been in charge for a very long time, and so it needs to learn how to become a team player with the rest of our faculties; it needs to learn how to slow down. I hear many people say that they've tried meditation, and that it's not for them because their mind takes them away from the breath and the stillness. They can't sit still, so they give up. If you happen to be one of these people, consider that your busy mind is actually functioning like this all the time and that the stillness of your meditation is simply drawing your attention towards it. Stilling the mind is like strengthening a new muscle, and there are many good books and teachers out there to help you with that training.

For this exercise, you're in luck. While quieting the mind is helpful, it's not a dealbreaker because in a guided meditation we give the mind something to do. Guided meditation, a wellness practice that's scientifically proven to have benefits,[3] is a tool that engages your receptive imagination to activate and change the vibrations of your thoughts, emotions, and sensations. Receptive imagination is exactly what it sounds like, by resting into your body while you listen to your guide (me in this case), you are allowing the faculty of your imagination to receive the emotions, thoughts, sensations, and images that the narrative in the meditation guides you toward.

So, get comfortable, relax your shoulders, place your feet on the floor, and take a couple of deep breaths all the way down into your belly. We are soon going to begin. The first time you read this meditation, simply slow down your pace and notice your breath as you read. Stay curious, be open, and allow the images that are invoked to form in your mind. Allow your awareness to feel into the areas in your body that you are guided towards. You can also go online and try the audio version I've created (*earthhearthealing.ca*). Listening to the audio version with your eyes closed will make the experience even more powerful, and doing this meditation three times in one week will maximize the impact it has.

---

3   Alvin Powell, "When Science Meets Mindfulness," The Harvard Gazette (website), April 9, 2018, https://news.harvard.edu/gazette/story/2018/04/harvard-researchers-study-how-mindfulness-may-change-the-brain-in-depressed-patients/

A Meditation to Activate your Divine Inner Child

Take a big inhale, and a big exhale. Focus on straightening your spine. You can imagine a string connecting to the top of your head that is gently being tugged toward the ceiling. Imagine the sensation of a light tug at the top of your head, and allow your spine to elongate. Now, imagine your sit bones (the bottom portion of your hip bones that are touching the seat) sinking into the chair, or the couch, or the floor and allow your spine to elongate even more. Roll your shoulders back and down and start to focus on your breath. Inhale and exhale. From here, send your breath all the way down through your core and down through your central channel. Located just in front of your spine, your central channel is the main energetic pathway connecting you to heaven and earth. As you travel down your central channel with your breath, imagine it continuing to move down through your legs and out the bottoms of your feet. Let the breath flow out the bottoms of your feet by imagining little windows opening in your heels. Visualize your energy traveling down into the earth. Allow it to form into the roots of a tree, or a rope, or a chain. Send your energy all the way down into the center of the earth, past the rock and the layers of soil, until you meet the crystalline core of the planet—a crystalline sphere of energy that connects you to the life force and healing emanations of earth's essence.

Feel, sense, imagine yourself there in the center of the earth, and visualize wrapping your energetic chain, light cord, or roots of your tree around the central crystalline core. You are now connecting your essence to the essence of the earth. Spend some time here. Once you can feel, sense, and imagine your connection, bring your energy back up through the earth, and allow the earth energy to come up through the earth too.

Imagine the little windows in your feet opening up to allow this energy to flow back in, breathe it up through your legs, allow it to fill your hips, and let it fill your abdomen. With the breath, take a big inhale and exhale, and once you reach your heart center, allow the energy of your consciousness and the earth's essence to sink in and soften. Inhale and exhale. Inhale and exhale. Inhale and exhale. Become familiar with your sacred heart space. From here, tune into your mind, and allow it to receive any impulses of thought, any visions or colors, and any felt sensations that connect you into this space in your heart. As you read these words, allow the space in your chest to deepen and expand. Your breath is responsible for moving you through your inner world, so allow your breath to breathe into the center of your chest.

From here, soften, and begin to imagine yourself as a young child, allow any memories to arise and let your imagination choose the age and choose the image. See if you can notice yourself appear. What are you wearing? What are you doing? What are you saying? What are you feeling? Are you happy or sad, excited or nervous, calm or energetic, wise or searching? If unpleasant memories arise, it's okay. Sometimes when we go deep into the heart, these types of memories come up because they hold emotions, which have yet to be processed. They arise because they are looking for resolution. For now, if those types of memories come, acknowledge them. Spend a moment creating a safe space for them to wait, and then tell them you'll come back. Then kindly place those memories aside for another date. Now call forth the magical and divine inner child who is there. Imagine yourself appearing as when you were first born into this world. See the curiosity and the joy that accompanied you as you looked out at this planet and the world of your childhood in those early years of life. Connect into the sensory experience of this and see if you can then hear your own laughter. Hear the essence of your own inner child, and as you do, take a look into his or her eyes. What do you notice? Can you find the purity, joy, and the innate self-love that emanates from this space of just being alive? Ask to find your inner joy for being alive. Inhale and exhale.

Spend some breaths here and let things evolve. Let your imagination receive what your inner child is doing. Where is your inner child at this moment as they express their innate joy and bliss? Notice what movements or activities they are partaking in naturally. Are they drawing, or dancing, or playing outside? Allow your inner child to create, move, be, dance, and allow the space they are in to expand with safety and bliss. Bring the experience closer to you. What smells do you notice? Inhale and exhale, and allow the innate feeling of love and joy to expand through your heart space now, in the present moment. As you focus on connecting your inner space to your outer space in the center of your chest, notice if there are any messages that are coming forth from this beautiful being that you are. Allow any messages of wisdom that may help you on your journey to arise at this moment. Breathe and invite yourself to remember the simplicity that existed before the outer world took form. Breathe and come back to the pulse of love that exists underneath our experiences at all times.

Invite your heart to open to the archetypal frequency of joy, bliss, magic, and purity that connects you to your soul and ask to feel your essence as it was before you stepped into life's outward play. While you're here in your inner imagination, it's time to acknowledge your divine inner child. Give him or her a hug, a nod, or a message of gratitude. Say "thank you" as they continue to play and explore. Then, if it feels right for you—allow their essence to light up and grow and pierce through all the cells in your body. Imagine every cell in your body filling up with the loving vibration of your divine inner child. Inhale and exhale. Breathe into your heart and know that you are loved. Allow a smile to form with your lips. Inhale and exhale and spend some time here—as long as you'd like.

Then, when you are ready, it's time to come back. Take another breath and imagine it reaching the outer edges of your body. Notice your skin as it meets the fabric of your clothes, begin to wiggle your fingers and toes, inhale and exhale, open your eyes, and come back.

Take a pause.

So . . . how was your inner journey? Could you feel a connection? Any insights? Any revelations? I had you do this exercise because it lays the foundation for the rest of the book, as I don't want you to just take my word for things. I'd like you to have a personal experience, which supports your inner transformation. Now is the time to do a little inquiry. What are the qualities inherent in your happy inner child? Innocence, laughter, spontaneity . . . go ahead and add a few of your own to the list. It's important to contemplate this because if you are someone who is experiencing Alzheimer's in a family member, illness in your life, would like to experience healing, or are just someone who is curious about spirituality, then this is the vibrational doorway that will allow your soul to become part of your journey.

Take this as your spiritual prescription because to continue with your training in the next couple chapters, you'll require this insight. The more you let the experience of knowing your divine inner child saturate your experience, the more opportunity it has to transform into wisdom. The divine and magical inner child is your soul's essence merging with your human nature, and all of us who are human have it. If you are someone who hasn't felt it yet and want to, know that energetic alchemy is like creating a line in the sand while the waves come in—we need to keep deepening the line for it to stick. So, keep exploring with curiosity because this is where your foundation of self-love comes from. See if you can take off the adulting hat for a little while and explore the world of your inner child. See if you can take *little you* by the hand and invite them to come along as your guest of honor.

In the next couple of days, take some time in service of contemplation and experimentation. You can journal, take a walk, or do what you always do and see if you can do it in a new way from the inside out. For this window in time to merge with your day-to-day activities, see if you can step in closer to yourself to allow this new essence of love and joy into more parts of your life; where the only thing that this joy and love is connected to is your breath. Through the eyes of your divine inner child practice living the simple joy of just being alive.

***

From our souls' point of view, dis-ease is the reflection of an imbalance in our natural state, wellness, and health. If that is so, then it's the purity of our inner child who connects us most closely to presence and the zero-point energetic of our soul that is capable of emanating pure potential. If we infuse that potential with the desire for truth, health, and well-being, that's when we'll be able to receive the guidance that we need to walk our own healing journey. The psyche of the divine inner child naturally knows what is good for us and what isn't, and in that sense he or she is immensely wise beyond their years. This is the part of you that will fuel your unraveling, and the part of you that will reveal the work that needs to be done.

When I started to explore the healing arts, I got off the mainstream train and left my original dreams behind because it didn't seem to align with how happy I was feeling. I also found, through experience, that we create our own reality and at that time was introduced to the idea that we create our own illness. And although I still think this is half true, I've also learned something new: the darkness that exists in the power holding tiers of our current world is a powerful force. So, even though it's our job to take responsibility for our actions, from a soul level, there are some odds that have been stacked against us for quite some time.

The dynamics between the darkness and the light in the current paradigm script that we live in, have been written in a way where the light has lost its primary role as the leading character because the dark has taken control through cunning deceit. Also, we don't see this imbalance in an obvious way because our limitations are often set by a glass ceiling. For each one of us, it means that our divine inner child, and by affiliation our soul (the version of us who knows that we are the co-creators of our own life), has taken the back seat. As a collective, we have given our power away to authority without doing enough homework. But, this is where things get exciting for you. The difference for you, as an adult with an active divine inner child, is you now have the required components for a formula that has the capacity to rewrite your current script (organically and over time).

Chapter Eight:
Your Subtle
Anatomy

I consider myself a renegade of the mainstream. In my heart, I believe that we are entering a new stage of evolution in the collective consciousness of our species. There is a part of me who holds a vision of that future, and another part of me who is committed to sharing that vision. It's a vision of the new paradigm, and whether it takes two years, two decades, or two centuries, we will grow in a way that removes the need for the existence of illness because its role as a teacher will have served its purpose. For humanity, planet earth can be considered a school, and that school is evolving into a space where heart-centered relating can become the new normal. A place where we are connected to our souls, where we are sovereign, and where the energy of our individual existence is fueled by our soul energy pouring out into the world around us for our enjoyment through service. Rather than a society where control and polarity fuel our learning, creativity, personal sovereignty, transparency, and **natural law** can become our dominant template. We will have the opportunity to experience living in a more enlightened way. This brand new collective template won't come from a top-down system that is implemented for us, either. It will come from each one of us choosing to do the work of our personal evolution from the inside out, and how we will create that in our lives is up to us to discover.

In the previous chapter, I said that the difference between then and now on this journey of healing, is that now you are an adult *and* a child. Having both of these perspectives active, has the capacity to rewrite your personal script through love. It's the child in you who holds the magic that can alchemize all experiences, and it's your adult self who will be the one to **transmute** that energy by implementing the required changes. You didn't think I was telling you to let your four-year-old drive the car or run the team at work, did you? I am not saying that. What I am saying is that your divine inner child should be your main consultant. They are the one who will guide you and help you to make the choices that are in alignment with your soul. Your divine inner child naturally follows the new paradigm's template, and it will become inherent within when you align yourself with goodness. No one is excluded who desires this path, either, and that's why I love teaching it. It's like honey for the heart.

***

Now that your soul is awakening, and if you'd like to continue cultivating this awakening, your next task will be to listen and to align yourself with it. Aligning your life with the goodness of your true nature, means that anything that is not in alignment with that goodness or balance will need to be integrated and released (organically and over time). This is where your personal healing work will be. You will be making new choices, and for that, you'll need a new template to support you. That's why this chapter is about the anatomy of your auric field, and how its layers participate in creating your life experience. Having an interest in your aura can benefit many areas of your life, and here in this book it will be with a focus on how to remove the denser parts of your unconscious programming that is causing you to create imbalance and pain. These parts are probably trauma-based programs (a function of the old matrix) that are no longer in alignment with your soul.

The Foundations of Your Subtle Anatomy

When you are given something to read that is being presented as science (like this manual for example), consider that the definition of science is this: *the intellectual and practical activity encompassing the systematic study of the structure and behavior of the physical and natural world through observation and experiment.*[1] Scientific information that has been written down as fact in a book, first came forward from a soul, or many souls, who were in observation and experimentation mode. They formed a hypothesis, then carried out tests on that hypothesis, and they then saw how many times the same result occurred. This is the same process you follow to understand the truths in your inner world too. As children, scientific discovery was natural to our growth, and we can recreate this same *naturalness* in our experience at any time. Consider physicist Pascual Jordan who said that, "Observations not only disturb what has to be measured, they produce it . . . We compel [a quantum particle] to assume a definite position."[2] In other words Jordan said, "We ourselves produce the results of the measurements."[3] What this means to me is that human consciousness produces the theory, and

1   "Science," Oxford Lexico (website), accessed February 07, 2021, https://www.lexico.com/definition/science.

2   Max Jammer, *The Philosophy of Quantum Mechanics: The Interpretations of Quantum Mechanics in Historical Perspectives* (New York: John Wiley, 1974), 161.

3   Pascual Jordan, "Quantenphysikalische Bemerkungen zur Biologie und Psychologie," *Erkenntnis, 4* (1934): 215–232, https://www.jstor.org/stable/20011714.

by focusing our thoughts on that theory while we carry out the required action, we also create its results. By being conscious with our actions, we have an influence on what we are creating, and we create all the time. As each psychic being is unique, the theories they create and the results they find will be unique to them. In other words, it means that we are all part scientist and that we can loosen our bonds on the status quo and acknowledge the potential we have to create new and healthier systems. We are the co-creators of this reality, and the collective beliefs we have are because we have a collective inner garden (or collective subconscious). You might be surprised to find that these collective beliefs are more malleable than you'd expect.

That's my introduction on science and the mind; have you ever considered science and the heart? Were you ever taught to hold your hands to your organs to get to know them personally when you learned human biology in school? Or to love the cells that create your nose? Love is the component of our expression that does the deeper relating in relationships. We get to know other people, new ideas, new experiences, and the unique aspects of ourselves more deeply through the art of loving. There is a lot of learning that can happen through love, and just like you might support a small child in their development, we can support the healing and growth of a particular organ or area of the body when we give them our love too.

So, take a breath. Stay curious as you read because *you* are the one creating these ideas in your experience while you place your focus on my words. In its most authentic form, science related to our light bodies should stay malleable because consciousness is ever evolving and transforming. There is wisdom in the phrase that says, "The only thing constant is change." It's just my suggestion, but do less of seeing this next bit of data as words on a page, and more like you are experiencing a new dimension of your awareness, which you can explore through your inner science geek and through love.

High Sense Perception (HSP)[4] / *Extra-Sensory Perception (ESP)*[5] / *Subtle Sense Perception:* I introduced this capability as subtle sense perception in chapter three because this title feels the most relatable to me, yet the more common name for this capacity is High Sense Perception (HSP), and in other circles it goes by the name Extra-Sensory Perception (ESP). Just like you have your five senses of hearing, smell, taste, touch, and sight to navigate the physical world, you also have high sense perception to navigate the non-physical world of subtle energy that you live in. In chapter six, I introduced you to your receptive imagination, but that's just the tip of the iceberg when it comes to your potential. As far as HSP is concerned, there are five generally accepted categories. They are the basics and depending on the research you do you may find more, such as the ability to affect weather patterns or to speak with the animal kingdom.

Clairvoyance is the ability to see subtle energy in the outside world, like the aura, or the ability to see things in your internal world, like events and images without being physically present to them. This type of internal seeing can interpret information that comes from the past, future, or even from another dimension of reality. People who experience clairvoyance see with their mind's eye *or* third eye, and this inner vision is connected to the pineal gland in the mind.

---

4   Elaine Aron, *The Highly Sensitive Person: Maximizing Performance and Controlling Stress.* New York: Carol Publishing Group, 1996.

5   Noel Sheehy, Antony J. Chapman, and Wendy A. Conroy, *Biographical Dictionary of Psychology* (London: Routledge, 2016), 409.

Clairsentience is the ability to sense energy through feeling. It most typically becomes a heightened emotional awareness, but it is also the capacity to feel the essence of what you experience. Clairsentience is connected to the heart chakra.

Clairaudience is the ability to receive messages through inner hearing.

Claircognizance is a direct knowing of the truth.

Clairalience is the ability to receive psychic impressions through smell.[6]

HSP is natural to the human body; it's innate, but it's not always turned on. However, these days it is becoming more common for children to have this activated from birth. While in adults, turning it on requires a desire to do so, and then some earnest effort. When you take the time to cultivate your HSP it will likely evolve in subtle increments, and gives you the ability to be more attuned to your environment. It's also the tool that allows you to interact with your aura in order to pull up old programs. It gives you a new level of awareness, and the capability to move information that's been stored in your inner self (what is in your subconscious and below your awareness), into the awareness of your outer self for you to heal.

At this particular time in our human history, in congruence with our species becoming more conscious, it's expected that it will become more common for people to be aware of their auras. If this is happening for you already, you may notice that you are becoming more sensitive to your environment. Experiences where you used to feel content may now feel irritating, or if you are in an environment that is on purpose for your soul, you may

6   Laurie Barraco, *Psychic Development 101: Easily Tap into Your Natural Psychic Abilities* (Independently Published, 2019), 15-17.

find your experiences becoming more blissful. It's commonly accepted that between fifteen and twenty percent of the population are already *highly sensitive people*,[7] so if you're not one yourself, chances are you'll know somebody who is.

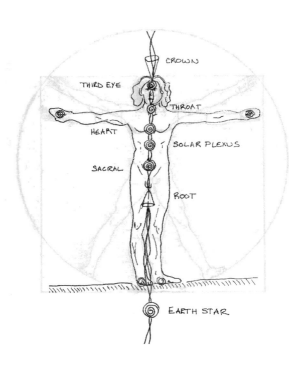

THE CHAKRAS

---

7   Aron, *The Highly Sensitive Person.*

The Aura [8] / *Light Bodies* / *Biofield* [9]*:* Your aura is your moving map, and a holistic view of how your soul's essence interfaces with the rest of your physical body. It also brings locality to the unique screens through which we each see life; we really are *in our own bubble* in that sense. Becoming aware of the layers of your auric field is like receiving a personal copy of your human manual. It means that you are being given more governance over yourself, and because you are now more aware, it also means that you'll have some work to do in cleaning out your inner garden. Inside your field you have seven layers of information and seven main chakras that connect into those layers to transfer energy. Yet, even this basic statement varies among specialists because the more expanded we get in our awareness, the more chakras and layers of our field we can activate and expand into.

Enlightenment of the physical body is all about light quotient, and as an incarnated soul and developing psychic being, that light quotient will continue to expand outward and inward through your auric field the more that you grow. Relative to the purpose of this book, knowing the basics such as your central channel, your seven chakras, the earth star chakra (which we connected to in the meditation exercise), and the five lower layers of your auric field, will do you just fine. Most explanations will be in this chapter, while some will be in the next, and as we move through them I invite you to gently place your hand onto the area of your body you are reading about and connect using your subtle senses.

8   C.W. Leadbeater, *The Chakras*. London: Theosophical Publishing House, 1975.

9   Beverly Rubik et al., "Biofield Science and Healing: History, Terminology, and Concepts, *Global Advances in Health and Medicine, 4* (November, 2015): 8-14, https://doi.org/10.7453/gahmj.2015.038.suppl

The Central Channel: Located just in front of your physical spine, this is your main channel of spiraling energy that brings life force or **prana** into and out of your body, and to and from its different areas. Your central channel runs energy in two directions, down from the heavens connecting you to the wisdom of the cosmos, and up from the earth connecting you to the life-affirming energies of mother earth. It is the primary support system of your energetic anatomy just like your backbone is the primary support for your skeletal system. All seven of your chakras connect into your central channel to share information and transfer energy.

The Seven Chakras[10]: Each chakra is a cone-shaped spiraling vortex of energy that links and transfers energy to a gland in your body. They act as the bridge between what is physical and nonphysical, and between what is conscious and what is unconscious in your personal world. Their purpose is to input nonphysical energy into your system, like sound, color, psychic thought, or data through technology, so that you may incorporate them into your physical experience. The seven chakras also output these same non-physical energies, so that you can share and relate to the world around you. Just as I introduced them in chapter two, each chakra has a corresponding color and wavelength, and each is responsible for managing a particular component of your psychology related to the different areas of your life.

The Root Chakra: Your first chakra is located at the base of your spine and points down toward the ground. It is connected to your adrenal glands, and regulates your sense of survival. It is responsible for everything that has to do with safety, family, financial stability, and belonging.

---

10   Barbara Ann Brennan, *Hands of Light: A Guide to Healing Through the Human Energy Field* (Toronto: Bantam Books, 1993) 43.

Governed by the earth element, its vibration creates the color red.

The Sacral Chakra: Your second chakra is located just below the belly button and has two vortexes: one that emanates outward in front of you and one that emanates outward behind you. Its domain is pleasure and it connects to your ovaries or gonads (depending on your gender). It is responsible for everything in your life that has to do with sexuality, creativity, sensuality, and nurturance. Governed by the element of water, its vibration creates the color orange.

The Solar Plexus Chakra: Your third chakra is located just below the rib cage in the center of your body and has two vortexes: one that emanates outward in front of you and one that emanates outward behind you. The gland it connects to is your pancreas, and its domain is your personal identity. It is responsible for your sense of self, your self-esteem, and your metabolism. Governed by the element of fire, its vibration creates the color yellow.

The Heart Chakra / The Subtle Heart: Your fourth chakra is located in the center of your chest and has two vortexes: one that emanates outward in front of you and one that emanates outward behind you. Connected to your thymus gland, it is responsible for your relationships, love, healing, compassion, forgiveness, and balance. It vibrates with the color green if it's healthy and open, or pink if it's in the process of healing (meaning unifying pieces which are separate), and the element by which it's governed is air.

The Throat Chakra: Your fifth chakra emanates out from the front and back of your neck. Connected to your thyroid gland, your throat chakra is responsible for allowing you to express your truth, whether it's through voice, song, art, dance, a job you love, a family you love, or a dream you have. Governed by sound, its vibration creates the color blue.

The Third Eye Chakra: Your sixth chakra is located in the center of your forehead, and has a vortex of energy that emanates out through the front and back of your head. Connected to your pineal gland, this is where duality becomes unified and where you cease to see life through polarity. It's responsible for visioning your dreams, your intellect, your imagination, and your wisdom; making sense of the energies that you input into your system and allowing you to understand them. Governed by light, its vibration creates the color violet.

The Crown Chakra: Your seventh chakra is located at the top of your head and points up toward the sky. Connected to your pituitary gland, when it's open it allows you to connect with other dimensions of reality and to a sense of unity with life. Responsible for transcendence and governed by consciousness, its inherent vibration is white.[11]

Your seven chakras are connected to the seven layers in your auric field, and they connect in a similar way as A7 and C4 connect in the game Battleship. But instead of finding a ship in its location, what you'll find is an interface where energy can be transferred. Chakra wellness is reflected in the qualities of openness, balance, and alignment, while chakra unwellness is reflected in the qualities of blockages, imbalance, and misdirection. Healing them is a holistic transformation, and once you are aware they exist their movement towards healing is innate. It means that since you've activated your soul, your natural guidance will become activated as well, while implementing

11   Anodea Judith, *Wheels of Life: A User's Guide to the Chakra System.* St. Paul: Llewellyn Publications, 2016.

the changes that your guidance suggests will be part of your earnest effort. A soul-led life starts with learning to become your own best friend, and at this point in time in our collective story, some of the programs we were given are getting in the way of that.

A Code / *Program:* is constructed from a belief, an emotion, and a physical sensation in your body. Correspondingly, the third layer of your field is your mental body, the second layer is your emotional body, and the first layer is your etheric body. How we experience our reality is a reflection of, and a co-creation with the vibrational information that we contain in our earth-suit and these are the layers of your energy field that are responsible for everything that has to do with earth-life and your constructed reality.

Once you activate the inner navigation system of our soul-self, through the archetype of your divine inner child, those programs that are not in alignment with your highest potential for a healthy life will organically begin to reveal themselves. In other words, any program that is not in alignment with how you would treat a small joyful child (you), will naturally show up to be worked on. However, not all of the programs you have been given will be negative, some of them hold gifts. What's important will be taking the time to read what programs are creating your experience, so that you can learn from the lessons that are harming you causing them to dismantle, and expand into or create new ones that will bring you joy.

Earth Star Chakra: Before we begin to discuss how to deconstruct our harmful programs, it is helpful to have cultivated some *inner strengths*, or to have anchors in other areas of your life that you can lean on for support (these can be people, activities, a personal practice, and so on). One of the best anchors that I know of is mother earth, and that's where a connection to the earth star chakra becomes helpful to your well-being. The earth is one of our most beloved teachers and has a constructed reality which is highly conscious, healthy, and harmonizes with those who live upon her. For example, how the trees look and the oceans move are archetypal energies that we can appreciate, honor, and feel as though we are part of it.

Anchoring to the earth is an experiential part of the new paradigm template, and essential in the guided meditation to meet your inner divine child. That is why I first had you connect with the earth. If you continue to practice grounding your soul energy, eventually it will be your trauma-based relational programs that will come forward to be deconstructed. That's because just like Mother Mary, Doña María, and Mirra Alfassa teach, the earth's vibration is that of unconditional love and if you are in resonance with her, you'll learn how to love unconditionally too. Learning and practicing unconditional love, means that you'll be learning a new way to relate to others, to the other kingdoms on our planet, and most importantly with this new skill, you'll be learning a new way to relate to yourself.

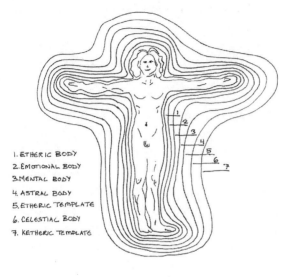

1. ETHERIC BODY
2. EMOTIONAL BODY
3. MENTAL BODY
4. ASTRAL BODY
5. ETHERIC TEMPLATE
6. CELESTIAL BODY
7. KETHERIC TEMPLATE

THE AURA

The Mental Body [12] / *Third Layer of Your Aura* / *Your Beliefs:* Our present society is one that operates strongly in the mind. However, not all of us who are in society fall into this category. For example, the consciousness of dancers and athletes lives strongly in the body, while for caregivers it may live strongly in the heart. Our society is one designed to place value, respect, and a sense of authority in those individuals who express their consciousnesses through intellect because our educational system is designed this way. Those who can think broadly, creatively, and systematically with conviction can excel. We also do the things we do, and stay the places we stay by rationalizing our choices. Oftentimes it's also the mind

12   Brennan, *Hands of Light,* 50.

that keeps us in situations that are no longer healthy for us. What most people are unaware of is that these thoughts exist not only in the mind, but also in the third layer of the energy field.

Located approximately three to eight inches from the body,[13] this layer of our field is composed of rigid and structural lines of vibrating light. It is created by what you think about, and is then formed from what you know and what you believe to be true. A strong and healthy mental body appears lit up in bright yellow with lots of energy moving through it, and interprets its environment based on the data it has already stored. A strong mental body is great if you are on purpose in the reality you live in, while if you find yourself on the healing journey, it may require changing some of those beliefs, which means deconstructing them from their root.

Here's an analogy. The mental body is like an exquisite sculpture, and one that is well developed is like having the ability to see from different vantage points of that sculpture (and in more or less detail, depending on where you are standing). A strong mental body would be able to make connections, and see the bigger picture from different angles, just like how a sculpture is three-dimensional, but appears two-dimensional until you begin to walk around it. Thinking causes the lines of light in your aura to illuminate and activate, and the more information about a certain subject you have, the more pathways there are, and the more thoughts there will be. Strengthening the current vibration in your mental field, which is much of what happens when you specialize in a subject, means that the mind will create more deductions, connections, explanations, and points of view from the same root belief(s). Yet, no matter

13   Brennan, *Hands of Light,* 50.

which way you continue to hone your craft, or if the sculpture gets more exquisite, it will stay made out of the same material. Deconstructing a belief is like choosing to change the sculpture's material or reconstruct your inner light.

To give you an example of what I'm talking about, I'm going to share another story with you, and it takes us back to my first Vipassana retreat. On my way back home from this life-changing experience, I found myself sitting in the Delhi Airport totally freaking out. I had taken everything I learned there straight to heart (which included not eating meat), and in that moment I was experiencing a *gut-gurgling* level of hunger. As I searched for a meal that met the requirements of my new diet, what I found was a mushroom sandwich—which I then bought, and eagerly opened out of its wrapper. As I sat there at a little table in the middle of a bustling airport, about to eat my Vipassana-friendly sandwich, I had a realization. I realized that the table was only vibrating energy, the chair was only vibrating energy, I was only a bubble of vibrating energy . . . and so was the mushroom sandwich. Solidity vanished and it hit me in such a hard and fast experiential way that I proceeded to lose my footing. What I experienced, as I sat there on my vibrating chair eating my vibrating mushroom sandwich, was an ego death. Something that happens when not just your mind, but the whole of you, from a powerful pulse that has emanated from your soul, asks you to change from the root. A demolition was spontaneously occurring and the material of my sculpture was changing.

The mental layer is the most superficial layer of programming, and in therapy when these thoughts pertain to our sense of self, we call them *our story*. Our stories are composed of our conscious beliefs, while our unconscious beliefs are those that lay their foundations. Unconscious beliefs are thoughts we've thought enough times during a certain period, that our mind has placed them into our sub-conscious awareness or locked away due to trauma, and if you've not yet discovered them they will feel like ultimate truths. On the one hand, this is an amazing capability to have, as we are then able to live the day to day with ease, while the danger in it is that once we stop thinking those thoughts consciously, they are just that, unconscious. If those unconscious beliefs are negative, they'll cause you to have negative life experiences, and if you've outgrown them, those experiences will block, deepen, and weaken the joyful pulse and wisdom of your soul.

The Emotional Body[14] / *Second Layer of Your Field* / *Your Instinctual Emotions:* Your emotional body is where your gut instincts and emotions are held, and the next step in analyzing a program is to look at the emotion(s) behind the beliefs you are studying. For example, a healthy connection between a belief and an emotion would be when intellect connects to passion, or caretaking connects to a loving devotion that fills you up. While an unhealthy connection would be when an intimate relationship connects to abandonment or abuse. When you say something with love, passion, hatred, or sadness, the words will carry more of a charge because your emotions are what are fueling them; they are e-motions *or* energy in motion.[15]

This layer is located one to three inches from the body.[16] In contrast to the structural nature of the third layer of your field, the second layer is fluid, like the clouds and like the ocean. Emotional energy can express through all of your chakras, but since this is a book on energy

14   Brennan, *Hands of Light,* 50.
15   *E-Motion*, written and directed by Frazer Bailey, executive producer Justin Lyon (Australia: Play Pictures). Documentary released 2014 in the United States, 87:00, https://www.e-motionthemovie.com/
16   Brennan, *Hands of Light,* 50.

healing, know that if you express these instinctual emotions through your heart (which we'll get to discussing later), you will have the ability to learn their lessons, which will be what transforms them into a more positive and aligned expression. The natural function of emotions is to express them without harmful action, and if they are negative you can learn the art of expressing them without action or **projection**, while still acknowledging what they are telling you—the truth of how your soul is feeling about a situation, or if you are clearing out an old story from the past, how you were feeling at that time. Some techniques to accomplish this are things like screaming into a pillow with all your might when you are feeling rageful to verbally reinstate your boundaries, or writing your sadness into a letter, learning from it through self-reflection, and then burning that letter to symbolize your earnest desire for transformation and closure. Your emotional patterns can also be sophisticated, and there will likely be many emotive cues before you reach a train wreck in your life. So, during the process of excavation, acknowledging and separating the different layers (ie. sadness, anger, guilt, joy, contentment) will be what helps you to release them.

Holding in your emotions is the opposite of health because emotions are innately meant to be expressed in order to be metabolized. As a result of growing up in a mind-based society, however, many of us have been raised to hold our emotions. What happens to us over time is this: the free flowing energy in motion will densify and create blockages as we repeatedly decide to repress what those emotions are cueing us to do. Repression creates a slow descent into more restrictive ways of thinking, and a backlog of emotional energy is akin to filling rooms in your home until they are so full that you feel you must then close the doors in order to contain what's inside. Eventually you'll end up only living in a room of 200 square feet, rather than your house of 2000 square feet. Repressed emotions will mix, grey out, and restrict the openness of your curiosity, and how you are feeling moment to moment can then turn into confusion, anxiety, or depression. Eventually this way of living will replace the precision of your emotional awareness as you'll no longer be able to make sense of what your inner self is telling you. If you are successful in repressing your feelings out of your awareness, you might stop feeling them altogether, but emotional energy never really leaves unless it's outwardly expressed or inwardly metabolized. Instead, your feelings get pushed in the opposite direction, and create an impression in the first layer of your field. The denser they become, the more you might start feeling that *chronic pain* in your lower back or shoulders as your physical body begins to offer its reflection.

The second layer of the auric field moves the energy that is connected to your pleasures and pains in life, and as a child these fundamental connections are made between emotion and thought based on your unique predisposition. Western society hasn't fully understood the power of emotions connected to a loving heart, and so dogmatic programming has become common. **Dogma** gets created in our auric field as children when we aren't given the opportunity to reflect on how we feel about the information that we were given. Learning in this way creates the potential for bonds to be formed between beliefs and emotions that aren't in alignment with the soul.

When we reactivate our soul-self, the undoing of this dogmatic programming is what will cause most ego deaths, and because many of us have been taught to repress our emotions, re-experiencing their layers can be confusing and lengthy (for a time). The undoing of dogma is the breakdown between a belief and the emotion that held it in place and empowered it. In the process, our stories and beliefs don't disappear. Instead the emotional charge will disconnect, and the feeling of needing to express the old thought or belief will no longer have a force behind it. The old thought will then become like a factual memory, and once fully healed you'll be able to talk about that memory with curiosity and reflectivity instead of attachment or resistance.

The Etheric Body[17] / *First Layer of Your Field* / *Your Subtle Sensations:* This layer of your field is structural and the energetic blueprint for your physical cells. These lines of light create the highway that delivers nonphysical data to your cellular biology as you live your life. It permeates your body, and extends between one quarter to two inches from it.[18] Through the communication system of your **nadis** *or* **meridian lines**, and chakras, it is the layer that informs your physical structure of the changes that are happening in your mental, emotional, and spiritual fields. Without it, the matter that creates your physical body would have no connection to how you think and feel, and the physical matter itself—without a subtle blueprint to inform its specifications—would become like decentralized particles of stardust aimlessly floating around in the universe. And that's not an exaggeration, in fact, it was exactly how I was feeling back in the Delhi airport.

As I sat there alone contemplating my new vibrational reality, with a mushroom sandwich as my only companion, I was feeling as though on the verge of a spontaneous combustion. The thoughts in my head were: *what's happening to me? . . . what have I done? . . . am I becoming enlightened . . .* and, *what is the point of this existence?* As mental breakdowns usually include a sense of impending doom, I

17   Brennan, *Hands of Light,* 49.
18   Brennan, *Hands of Light,* 49.

felt that I needed more support than was currently at my disposal. So without any rhyme or reason, I got up from the place I was sitting, beelined to the small airport bookstore, and found guidance. There at eye level on the shelf staring back at me was something familiar: the book *Eat Pray Love,* there to save me for the second time. Instantly, I took the book in my hands, flipped it open without a thought, and landed on the very page that explained Vipassana as being an "ultra-orthodox, stripped-down, and very intensive Buddhist meditation technique, [and] the Extreme Sports version of transcendence."[19] I had no memory of ever reading these lines, nor any theoretical understanding of the subtle bodies at the time of my mushroom sandwich, and so these became the words that derailed my potential spontaneous combustion, and brought me back to a comforting reference point. With immense gratitude, I thanked Elizabeth Gilbert for her perfect words, and then I proceeded to carry on.

Vipassana is largely focused on training us to relate to our etheric template while in a meditative state. It teaches us to become aware of our natural tendency to attach to and resist life at the sensorial level, and to shift those energetic links by absolving imbalances through balance. The deepest part of our programming is the subtle sensations that we feel inside of our body and some examples of these subtle sensations are coolness, numbness, tingles, pulsating heat, and a sense of restriction or pressure. It's often the case that we have very little awareness of this layer of our being, and it's something that takes time to activate. That's why I'm such an advocate for Vipassana, it's my method of choice if you'd like a fast track to this layer of awakening. The course offered me the right environment consisting of silence and the temporary

---

19   Elizabeth Gilbert, *Eat, Pray, Love: One Woman's Search for Everything* (New York: Penguin Books Publishing PLC, 2006), 172.

elimination of my external world, in a time frame of ten days, and a modality that is said to be preserved in its original format straight from Buddha himself. As it relates to our programs, learning to access this layer of our field is like digging up a weed from its root, and makes us that much more effective in our own evolution.

It may also be comforting to know that the deconstruction of an old program that you carry doesn't have to come with the feeling of catastrophe that I felt the first time I went through an ego death. I am an extreme example. But, if you are feeling something similar to how I felt, know that you will make it through to the other side. You can embrace your experience as a literal *breakdown* of your mental energy (from its connection to a particular emotion), and soften into the insecurity of your experience knowing that it's natural to feel this way. Perhaps aim to focus on the sensorial experience of what you are going through, to make the transition less turbulent and more timely, and remember that things are simple before they are complex. Stay focused on your breath when things get stormy. Breath equals movement (through life), and this simple reminder will help you to navigate through your more difficult moments with presence.

On the other hand, if you have no experiential understanding of what I'm talking about, but still feel a resonance with this information, know that sincere intent is a powerful catalyst. So check in, and if it feels right for you, you can try this: take a big and natural inhale and exhale, and place your hand on your heart. Close your eyes (once you read to the end of the chapter), and with a sense of sincerity toward yourself and your soul, pledge that you are ready to start doing the work—it's best if you pledge with sincerity three times in a row.

Chapter Nine:
Enter Soldier Al

Your external environment is a direct reflection of your internal environment, is an esoteric principle related to the enlightened nature of the human being. We are the consciousness that creates, and the batteries that charge the reality we live in. Traditional society (or the present matrix), is currently disconnected from this knowledge because it's the way that our collective soul has chosen for us to learn. As a collective, we have chosen to incarnate into a matrix that teaches us through separation, through ego, and through a less powerful perception of who we are. However, this illusion causes us to live separated from our pain as well, which we have helped to co-create. In the material and mind-based culture of the present, we don't usually become aware of the pain we carry until we see it manifest physically. Yet, before it shows up in our body, it will have a more subtle expression or in other words a first program.

On a macro level, illness in action is expressed through experiences like war and corporate control, and on a micro level, it is expressed through our various forms of disease. What might be new for you, is to consider that illness is a reflection of programs that hold repressed pain, and that holding onto that pain is a collective choice, and not something that is innate to the soul. These illnesses that are created through our unconscious programming, are then reflected back to us as imbalances within our personal world; the one that was bestowed upon our soul to care take, manifest, and learn through. When we grow to embrace the power in this new knowledge, it then becomes important to understand our shadows. In other words, what we don't yet know about ourselves and a field of exploration that is commonly known as shadow work.[1]

Energetically speaking, you learned that programs in the human experience consist of a mental, emotional, and subtle physical component. These three layers of our energy field relate to each other and create our unconscious drivers, and in a sense these layers also create our egoic nature. Meaning that our programs will directly influence how we see the world through our unique personalities (a personality, which by the way had been constructed from the alignment of the cosmos at the time of our birth . . . are you feeling magical yet?) Change a program and you change the way you see the world. To have been successful in changing one of your programs means that you have also learned its corresponding lesson. For example, while the concept of the answer key I spoke of in chapter one offered me the vision for a new destination, I still needed to live my own life experience in order to reach it. Through the lens of the soul, these new experiences excitingly become the hero's journey, and life is now staged to learn soul-based lessons. A good tip for getting yourself into the lesson learning frame of mind, is to also realize that you are the one who decides what lesson it is that you're

1   Connie Zweig and Jeremiah Abrams, *Meeting the Shadow: The Hidden Power of the Dark Side of Human Nature*. New York: G.P. Putnam's Sons, 1991.

learning, and that those lessons will appear when you are ready to learn them.

The Astral Body [2] / *Fourth Layer of Your Field* / *Your Relational Emotions:* Your astral body's primary connection is to your heart chakra, and a function of this layer is its ability to absolve programming in the lower three. Located one half to one foot from the body, this layer is cloud-like and emotional similar to the second layer of your field,[3] while it differs in the way that it relates to these emotions: through the heart rather than through instincts. Human beings are an exciting species for the soul to incarnate into because we have the ability to feel a very diverse spectrum of emotions, from the most hellish to the most angelic. That's why earth life can be painful at times, yet when we reconnect with our divine inner child, it creates a shift in our awareness and our comfortable resting point then becomes one of tangible goodness. This self-loving nature is what allows us to feel our deservedness to rest in higher love, and so we begin to fight for it.

One of the expressions in our current paradigm is that we can project our hurt onto others or into a story (even one that is very far away from us), and then feel it as separate from ourselves. Likewise we can also internalize our stories, so the pain that we feel will then appear isolated from the outside world. These ways of understanding pain are actually two sides of the same coin: internalized pain restricts the outward expression of who we are and gives our power away, while externalizing pain places us in a position of power over others in our psyches. Learning to live from a soul-centered heart, however, is like learning to see the coin as a whole. In doing this, we then have the

---

2   Barbara Ann Brennan, *Hands of Light: A Guide to Healing Through the Human Energy Field* (Toronto: Bantam Books, 1993) 51.

3   Brennan, *Hands of Light,* 51.

ability to hold that coin in the palm of our hand, allowing us the opportunity to then place it into our hearts. When this happens the pain can then be absolved through transparent relating, the release of emotions, and the humility that comes through us when we successfully learn the lessons that the hero's journey is offering. In the heart field, we will then know when we are not being authentic, and we will immediately feel the good and bad of our thoughts and actions. With this new sensitivity activated, we'll naturally desire to create a dynamic of feeling good in our outward expression towards ourselves and others.

If the heart chakra is emanating green we are expressing and thus in a co-creation mode; just like the dewy green grass on an early summer's morn, we are growing, doing, and expressing ourselves with the world around us through relationships. In the present matrix, many of us have been taught to be in co-creation mode conditionally. Meaning that we judge what is right and wrong before we offer our love. For example, we often love our spouses and children when they act in a way we approve, and then withhold that love when they don't. When we sink into the power of the heart the order of what's important to us changes, and the essence of those who are closest to us becomes more valuable than their actions, while right action is always the goal. We learn to keep our **core boundaries,** and also learn to see through eyes that value the wellbeing of others as they would like it to be. When we shift into the heart, harmonious action can then be taken through connected relating rather than through a more superficial sense of right and wrong, as we create our immediate worlds.

A heart that is emanating pink means it is healing, and it does this healing through resting in compassion. While passion is a creative driving force that comes through our second chakra, compassion is a unifying driving force that comes through our heart. Compassion is like the child of poetic joy and watchful wisdom, and is a particular lens of experience that linearity and rational thinking doesn't foster all that well. Compassion's gift is the loving ability to receive the truth exactly as it is, and not how we imagine or wish it to be. When we activate compassion as it pertains to our programs, we'll have the new ability to make conscious changes in our life, as compassion initiates the process of transmutation, which allows the energetic component of a program to transform into something new. In other words, compassion is the *being* required before the *doing*. In the old paradigm, we have created separation between us and the world around us on all levels, and to absolve the walls that this conditioning has created a healing heart is the golden ticket. Through the heart's teachings, we learn to relate to ourselves like our own best friend; we learn forgiveness, and through unity our pain no longer has the option to stay alive unconsciously in our inner gardens. A compassionate heart with the right personal boundaries, can lead us to a very happy life.

The Etheric Template [4] / *Fifth Layer of Your Field* / *Your Trauma-Free Template:* If your divine inner child is the one revealing to you the next steps of your deconstruction, your higher self (a vibration that holds a similar energetic to that of the answer key) is the one telling you what it is you are desiring to become. The fifth layer of your field is your trauma free original blueprint, the home of your higher self, and something that becomes helpful to access when we need direction. I remember a time in my life when I was in deep despair, and pretty drunk after coming home from a night on the town. Post break up and very sad, I was crying myself to sleep. Then, in a flash of vision, I saw a beautiful angel come

---

4   Brennan, *Hands of Light*, 52.

down in my mind's eye to tell me that everything was going to be okay. As she got closer, I began to cry even more because I noticed that she was me.

The template in your fifth layer is located one and a half to two feet from the body. Structural in nature,[5] it is the part of you that holds the holistic and healed vantage point of your incarnation. It shows you the fullness of whom you can be when you learn to love yourself (organically and over time). Let's say that both your etheric body and your etheric template are like an old Victorian mansion. In your etheric body, this mansion has been lived in, but also abandoned. It's been renovated and added to, while portions have also been demolished. It's had a long and dramatic life, and now lacks the vision required to transform it into a loving home once again. One of the people who own this property are off in search of a new place to live. Your etheric template exists on the other side of the self-love portal. This version of the Victorian mansion is in mint condition, and maintained through the loving energies of a generational care-taking and a structurally sound plan for the future. In this version, its owners are exactly where they want to be, and where friends and family want to be too.

The etheric template is found outside of you through the way that you interact with the world, just as it is found within you in your energy fields. To know its vision means that your fifth density self has become available to you! This is where your divine inner child is leading you when they guide you to transmute the pain that is holding you back from its experience. It's the expression of you if you were trauma free, whom with every step you take on the hero's journey you come closer to

5   Brennan, *Hands of Light,* 52.

becoming. Excitingly in our human evolution, it's where we are now able to go, and not just as individual souls on the path, but also as a collective.

***

If the mark of a good teacher is to practice what they preach, then in the case of a healer, it is to have experienced that which they are helping others to heal from. That's why the rest of this chapter explains how Alzheimer's disease began to show up in my inner world after my time with Ms. J had ended. Although I was only in my thirties and not showing symptoms, I was aware of the imbalances I had between my trauma-free template (as a child) and who I had become. Because one of the gifts of our divine inner child is that they have the ability to lead us to the programs we hold that are in violation of the sovereignty of our soul, and the vision they offer allows us to see those things in ourselves before they become physical. Their voice is the one that comes through those inner nudges that say not to take the job or stay in the relationship, or to speak up or create a new boundary. It is the voice of your empowered purity, and these are the types of doorways that will lead you to create healthier foundations.

To help you integrate what you've just learned, you can probably guess that we are going to take a more vibrational and holistic approach to Al's presence. We also have a spiritual puzzle piece in our back pocket that most data on Alzheimer's doesn't acknowledge, which gives a unique perspective. We know that to a soul experiencing the late stages of Alzheimer's disease, the body is no longer its permanent address. Why does this happen? What dynamic factors have been experienced by a living human soul that would direct them to split from their earthsuit, leaving them to live in two worlds? I took these questions with me on my deep dive, and before I share my journey of getting to know Al in my own life, I'd like to tell you more about why I love being a healer and the reason I spend much of my time in these deeper waters.

While awakening to the healing arts, I learned that I have the ability to highlight discordant programs. Once I realized this, highlighting them has become one of the most interesting parts of my life experience. I am the one looking for the needle in the haystack, while others are out enjoying a horseback ride in the field. I have an inner nature that likes to unify and balance with the world around me, and sometimes the needle in the haystack needs to be removed in order to achieve that. We are all capable of this inner precision, while for me it has become my joy.

Since before I can remember, the area around the front and back of my physical heart has felt numbed out, and as a child the hypochondriac in my imagination ran wild with reasons. When I voiced my concerns during routine checkups, the doctor would assure me that I was fine, and that the numbness was likely caused by tension in my muscles. "Perhaps I could see a specialist in that area," was their suggestion, and for some reason I never did. Numbed out parts of the body as they relate to the etheric body, are usually a way to mask the pain that's underneath and in my case, since the pain was something I had carried for my entire life, I had no memory of my initiation to this pain. Instead, it was just how I had always been.

When I entered the world of holistic healing, a devoted yoga practice and dedication to inner work allowed me to transform this area around my heart in a more holistic way. As a reflection of this work, my relationships with others have also become more honest and easeful because

I first learned to become more honest and easeful with myself. Then, when my journey gravitated towards energy healing, I learned that the pain I was experiencing could also be traced back to the etheric template that permeated my physical heart. I also became curious about the all-pervading and unexplainable blanket of thought that told me I needed to stay in hiding.

Investigative research into the nature of my condition heightened as I began this book and Al became my new best friend. Naturally, and even though he wasn't much of a talker, I allowed Al to reveal himself by focusing my receptive imagination on the area around my physical heart (a very adult way of saying that I spent time with my new imaginary friend). What were the results of our time spent together? I have come to understand that Al is stationed around my heart because I had asked him to. I did this asking many moons ago when I was only a child—I asked Al to protect me. Al is a silent, one-man task force, and I have come to know him fondly as my friend and devoted assistant, Soldier Al. I see him in my mind's eye like a Viking soldier, stationed in the snowy tundra, and standing guard at the doorway to the castle of my heart. It seems to be that Al has frozen my early childhood pain (and my first initiations into the trauma matrix), which, to a sensitive child, can be as innocent as a loud car driving by with no parent there to shield them, an authoritative parent yelling in a moment of stress or anger, or as devastating as the death of a parent or being born into war. In my case, Soldier Al showed up to protect me from feeling the pain, and as is typical with early childhood experiences, his existence dropped into my subconscious programming. I forgot about his arrival, carried on, and grew up.

In the divine inner child meditation, when I invited you to practice cultivating their essence, I did so by guiding you into the invocation of imagery, sound, emotionality, smells, and inner knowing. To learn more about Al, I used the very same technique, with a couple of minor alterations, as in this case, I didn't yet know where I was going. So, instead of following a script I let my breath and intuition be my guide. I set my intention to learn more about the numbness around my heart, and then I practiced becoming the witness to my internal world. With compassion in one hand and curiosity in the other, I placed my awareness and breath to the area around my heart in meditation, while in my outer life I used the framework that the layers of the aura offer to read between the lines of what I was living. I practiced living closer to myself.

The Energetic Program of Solder Al

The First Layer / *Subtle Sensations:* Numbness and tension around my heart and the back of my left shoulder blade. The sensorial experience of shielding and held strength.

The Second Layer / *Instinctual Emotions:* The practice of silence through stoicism and duty. The feeling of pushing down my true feelings, especially in service of convention. Many frozen emotions layered together.

The Third Layer / *Beliefs:* A soldier whose duty it is to protect my human heart. He emanates an unconscious belief that "the world is unsafe and that I need protecting."

The Fourth Layer / *Relational Emotions and Soul Lessons:* I am to remember the power and goodness that emanates from a soul-centered heart. My soul is desiring a new experience, and that means the completion and removal of an old program. My lesson is to learn how to love and be loved through an ever deepening authenticity.

The Fifth Layer / Trauma-Free Template: The expression of an open, loving, and feminine heart. My trauma-free template is a version of me who is no longer hiding behind closed doors.

When we experience the uprooting of an old program, it's our intention that activates a spiraling vortex of energy, which moves and lifts the necessary data through the loving God force within us. We allow our inner compass (or soul-self) to show us the pieces that we need to see, and how they are affecting us and the life we are living. It's a hand from the atman of our soul, scooping up all the aspects of a particular program as they express from all dimensions of our being. Just like we may have once desired the perfect home or dream career, our new conscious desire for more holistic wellness directs us toward the inner mechanisms of whom we really are so that we can remove the road blocks that inhibit us from becoming our best selves, and in the process we also create the enlightenment of our human vessel.

When and if you pull up an old program in your life, you are likely going to meet a character and a lesson. As you do this, I wonder . . . what type of teacher have you hired to share with you what's enclosed? For many people, the teacher that first shows up is this one: a voice of guilt, shame, and fear, that holds the remnants of an old school teacher or an authoritative father figure who's saying, "I am going to teach you a lesson because you are bad and you deserve it!" Or, perhaps the message is not so obvious, and only comes through the tone of their voice, or the pointing of a finger. I know this character too: they are a lead actor in the old paradigm's script. However, you are navigating new terrain now, and that teaching style is no longer helpful in leading you to your destination. So, with a big inhale and exhale, take some time to honor their efforts and with a sincere, "Thank you," you can now allow them to retire. If they are fussed about this, see if you can at least reduce their hours to part-time. Next, take some time to recreate your inner voice to sound more like this one: a kind and loving grandmother, who's passing you a warm drink as she speaks to you, "I am going to teach you a lesson, dear one . . . so that you can learn how to be the best version of a human that you can possibly be. I am going to teach you a lesson that is full of as much wisdom and knowledge that you can muster to take in because that is how much I love you, and that is how much I wish for you to know and to love yourself."

Your next assignment is to take a keen interest in your own life by honoring what shows up to be experienced. With your divine inner child leading the investigation, the voice of a loving grandmother as your new teacher, and the vision of whom you can become from your higher self as your final destination, you are now becoming the detective of you. Your personal file? Whatever you are experiencing right below your nose . . . and through the rest of your five senses . . . plus your HSP. Your personal file is your life exactly as it is at this moment, and taking an interest in your thoughts, feelings, subtle sensations, and now the insights and lessons that come through contemplation, will be what help you to expand the way in which you see it.

Chapter Ten:
Our Beginnings

Unconscious pain is the main culprit behind the imbalances that cause illness. In the same way, you could consider that once we become aware of the deeper layers of ourselves, it's the pain that we find there, which creates the barriers between a soul living in presence (permeating its energy through our body), and one that isn't. By recognizing illness through this new paradigm lens, all the blame, shame, sadness, and anger that we feel towards it will also diminish over time, as our soul-selves transform our psyche to support us in experiencing illness as a teacher. Contrary to the natural fear that most of us would feel toward a new diagnosis, illness is neutrally carrying out its job of reflecting the state of our consciousness (which has been calibrated over lifetimes) back to us.

Perhaps you're wondering how we have become so unconscious to our holistic reality. Well, like I said in chapter six, the world that we live in has conditioned us to be this way, and we have been programmed from childhood to function in it. However, we weren't born unconscious, and so I think it will be helpful to share with you how the auric field develops in childhood. We are capable of raising soul-centered humans, we just need to better understand how their subtle bodies grow.

With an effort to raise children who are attuned to their inner worlds, perhaps we could eliminate the need for Al's expression in our collective altogether.

The following theory on the energetic development of children comes to you from Barbara Brennan. She is a forerunner in the energy healing world, a former NASA scientist, and in her pioneering book, *Hands of Light,* she explains how our energy bodies develop in childhood.[1] Along with her theory, which is a popular one, I've infused some of my own insights as food for thought and to keep things fresh. Explained through the eyes of a soul as it incarnates into its earth-suit and egoic structure, my retelling of Brennan's theory begins pre-incarnation.

The Soul's Journey of Embodiment in Childhood

When a soul decides that it would like to incarnate, it's because it has chosen to take on its next assignment. It wants to be able to learn new things, and so it's chosen to forget everything it knows on a soul level; knowledge of beyond the veil, every incarnation it's ever had, universal wisdom, and so on. When a soul begins to incarnate, the first thing it does is create an energetic link between itself in the astral world and its newly fertilized egg. It's a dynamic that is very similar to that of a soul who is experiencing Alzheimer's, except that to live in two realms as a fetus is natural. As the fetus grows, the soul begins to feel an energetic pull towards matter and then in a flash of consciousness, much like the vision I had of my own soul energy zooming through a wormhole and into my mother's belly, the soul enters a little growing body inside its mother's womb, and begins the task of interfacing with its

---

1   Barbara Ann Brennan, *Hands of Light: A Guide to Healing Through the Human Energy Field* (Toronto: Bantam Books, 1993) 61.

newest physical vessel. Then the child is born. In the birth process the soul leaves the protection of its mother's flesh and becomes exposed to the atman field around it in a big way, and for everyone around, it's a moment of celebration and life on earth is again changed forever. A soul is born into this world, and to the earth it is a new note in the symphony of life birthed into form.

In the early months of life, the soul's job is to get used to the physical limitations of its new earth-suit, and it will still pop in and out through its crown chakra as it moves between realms and adjusts to the new density of earth. Even though it has a body, the soul has almost no sense of individuation because it is only at the beginning stages of forming its ego. This *almost* egoless state is reflected in an aura that is amorphous and underdeveloped, and the newly incarnated soul is assigned the task of growing its etheric body as the physical vessel also grows at a rapid rate.

Have you ever noticed how a young baby first learns to focus their eyes on the material world? As they learn to focus, their individuation is beginning to form through a feedback loop. The newly incarnated soul becomes acquainted with its new environment each time it's able to see into this reality, hear a noise, feel a sensation, or breathe. As the soul does this, it's breathing in the data that creates its aura. The human condition, relative to where the soul is born, downloads with every breath it takes, and it becomes a part of the web of light that is the human race.

Over the first three years of the soul's life, it has an umbilical cord of energy that connects it to its mother, and even if the souls are apart, they'll both still have a psychic sense of how the other is doing, and the mother will be able to feel this consciously. The soul's connection to its

122 | MARNIE O'FARRELL

mother is its primary support system, while it also benefits from the support and diversity of its immediate tribe.
Have you ever noticed how children easily find comfort
in the lap of a loved one, or cling to a parent when placed
in a new environment? That's partly because they hav-
en't developed the personal filter that protects them from
the world and are desiring protection. The energy field
of their caretakers acts as a shield until they can develop
their own.

Between the ages of two and seven years old, the soul is
focused on growing its sacral chakra and emotional body.
To learn to process experiences in an emotional way, it
will require a supportive environment, which is created by
those who love them. Then, through exploration and practice, the soul learns how to respond to life in a way that
is also consistent with its unique disposition as a psychic
being. When big emotions run through its new system,
the soul will need to complete each experience to have
governance over that emotion in the future. This expands
the calibration of the soul's nervous system to be able to
process a larger spectrum of energy in motion. As it integrates the large spectrum of emotions that life has to offer,
it must be supported to be successful.

In these early years of life, the way that the soul's
family members respond (or react) to life, will be the
early codes that are passed on to it through a process
called **co-regulation**[2] (something I'll go into more detail later in this chapter). During this stage of growth,
what the soul needs is a held space where it feels capable and safe, and one that allows its innate process to
innocently move through and integrate each new energy
as they come. As it moves through this process, it's a

2   Alan L. Sroufe, *Emotional Development: The Organiza-
tion of Emotional Life in the Early Years*. Cambridge: Cambridge
University Press, 2002.

good idea for the soul's caregivers to reflect to it the emotion it is feeling by verbalizing what's happening. This way their mental body can begin to create the appropriate connections for them, but it shouldn't be the main focus of their support at this time. To successfully integrate the bigger emotions that a soul in a young body is feeling, the caregivers' presence is what creates the training wheels. As caregivers, we can learn the art of creating boundaries while still allowing that soul to feel the fullness of their emotions through presence. Often isolating them (with a timeout) from those who can help them co-regulate the bigger emotions (like anger) when they are acting out, and before they have successfully learned to regulate their own emotions, will not set them up for a successful integration.

While its sacral chakra is developing, the soul also creates fantasy worlds, which allows its life-force to engage with the world around it. To the practicing youngster, its material possessions aid in this development and act as its training wheels for learning individuation. Before a child can play with others, it first learns how to be with itself. Through play, its toys become a literal extension of its life force as it learns to differentiate between itself and the world around it.

Then at age seven, when the mental body comes online more powerfully, a protective layer is created around each chakra, and the soul will feel much less vulnerable, and much more free. Its consciousness now begins to focus on the creation of its mental body, and the development of reason begins. By seven, the soul will have woven lines of gold light into the mental field around it, and the development of the soul's mental faculties are supported and enhanced through learning in school, as well as through play and fantasy (where most of its learning will take place). The soul's mental field taps into the archetypes in humanity; such as the princess, the superhero, or the doctor, and as it plays and integrates with the world where it was born, it learns where its affinities lie as they pertain to its life's journey.

In adolescence, the fourth layer of the energy field begins to develop: the soul's relational layer. In childhood, the soul experienced love with no separation from its family, while now it has a more fully developed sense of self. As this new layer activates, it sparks the capacity to love others in a more in-depth way through **eros**, which usually first appears on the scene as high school crushing. The soul begins to learn the art of relating; learning how to be what the person they adore wants while also desiring to stay true to its own individuality. The task of the soul then becomes a process of experiencing balance and extreme imbalance, as it adjusts to its desire for more autonomy and more intimacy within a more diverse scope of energies, and with someone who is not guaranteed to love them back. On a spiritual level, it could also be seen as learning its purpose and place within the whole, and then how to successfully relate to the world from those perspectives. It's the layer of the field that feels the fullest when it is giving and receiving love, and learning through living.

When childhood development is natural, our foundations will grow in an organic way that honors our unique soul. With phases of development that bleed into the next, we grow into our etheric body from zero to two, our emotional body from two to five, our mental body from five to seven and once we reach seven our foundational programs have been created. We develop filters over our chakras and at seven we begin to interact with the world through our own newly created individuation. As our mental bodies continue to develop, we strengthen in our capacity to reason and learn new information. Then in adolescence, our relational body comes online, and we experience a new desire to connect our emotional energy with someone who is outside our original family unit. We learn to connect more intimately through the heart, with an energy field that is separate from ours and our families.

***

When I was a child in elementary school, I wrote a poem called, "Why do we have war?" This was written for a Remembrance Day assignment. I remember how obvious it was to me that something between our innate human nature and how society was run didn't add up. How we got from A to B made no sense. When babies are born they smell soft and pure, and they do not have an innate fear of their surroundings. We come into this world with an open heart and a big spark in our eyes, and it's the honest task of our caregivers to keep it lit. I'm sure most people would agree, that although there are some adults who have been able to maintain their brightness, many are unsuccessful. Why as a society do we have trouble keeping our spark lit into adulthood? Instead, we have an elite group of bright stars, while the majority of us get weighted down with the stresses of the world.

If unconscious pain is the main culprit in disease, its sidekick would be trauma. Pair them up and you get unconscious pain from trauma. We have a mainstream human species who is unconscious to the power of its soul, and also to the sensitivity and spectrum of allowance, which is required to raise one properly. In the world of today, trauma has free reign, and we've normalized it as a part of the human experience because it is a part of our collective unconscious programming.

What is trauma exactly? Trauma is any experience for which we have been unable to remain present. For the soul, both good and bad experiences hold valuable lessons and learning opportunities, and so trauma is not found in the experience itself, but instead in the way that we process or fail to process through that experience. Something that we learn to do as children through co-regulation. To learn to feel the full spectrum of our emotions (from approximately two to five years old) we need parents who can stay present through a large spectrum of emotions in their own life, so that they can support us in staying present through our own. As a society we've been failing at this lesson, and I believe it's partly because we've given up our emotional sovereignty; we've been raised to reduce the importance of our emotions, and then lost our ability to have mastery over them.

Here's an example. Let's say there is a small two-year-old boy called Jim, who is crying because a toy has just been taken from him. His mother was cleaning up the playroom, as they were soon going to be leaving for daycare. When she takes his toy to put it away, he experiences a sense of shock and then a big emotion, and because his mother is rushing, she picks him up, apologizes to him as she is racing, and puts him in the car while he is still crying. Now they are driving and the rumble of the car takes the child's attention away from the pain that he feels, and he calms down. The mother eases, feeling relaxed now that her child is content again, but inside the child's energy field the pain has not been processed. Instead, it's been placed to the side as another moment has now taken the boy's attention. Because the child was not supported through his pain, the data of that unprocessed emotion drops into his inner being and becomes a small unconscious packet of energy in the lower layers of his energy field. Then the tactic of moving forward into the next moment without completing the painful experience is introduced, and assuming that the mother repeats this often (creating a pattern), a way of living will form to create one of the boy's foundational programs.

On the other hand, the key to having an experience that is negative but not traumatic, lies in our caregiver's ability to help us process through our emotions, and that is something that happens through presence. So, let's take the same example and make it a success! Jim is crying because his mother has taken a toy away from him, and instead of picking him up in a hurry and placing him in the car, she stops in her tracks once she hears him crying. Realizing her haste, she then stops to breathe and becomes present. With her intention, she tells her child that she is sorry for what she did, and that her actions were not OK. By resting in presence, she helps him to process his feelings. Her child's emotions are showing him that his soul (as it is human in this life) is not calibrated for such a forceful exchange. **Attunement** is required, and through it, his mother will find the right next step.[3] Maybe it's to leave her child right where he is, look into his eyes, breathe with him, and acknowledge his emotions as they move through them together. She may also use some soothing tones. Or, maybe he is so far away from his ability to regulate that she picks him up for a moment and lets him cry as she rocks him. Since the child is receiving support through co-regulation, an integrative solution is available for his emotional body to replicate and he calms down. Perhaps they are ten minutes late to their destination, yet the offering of an integrative pattern to the emotional body of the child has made a lifetime of difference.

In the first scenario, the child was innocently given a program that holds unconscious pain, and because it's unconscious, he may perpetuate that pain towards himself and others without knowing it in the future. While in the second scenario, the child was successful in completing

---

3   Daniel J. Siegel and Tina Payne Bryson, *The Power of Showing Up: How Parental Presence Shapes Who Our Kids Become and How Their Brains Get Wired.* New York: Ballantine Books, 2020.

the experience, so there is no unprocessed charge locked in his energy field. Instead, there is a program that says he's capable of staying present during a moment of pain because his mother was able to stay present and acknowledge it with him. Since he was given the opportunity to acknowledge the unpleasant feeling associated with this experience, he'll be aware of choosing more pleasant experiences for himself and others in the moments when they're possible in the future. In the second scenario, the child was given a program that honored his unique alignment to the purity and sensitivity of his soul's light.

Our ability to process through our experiences in a healthy way or in a way that creates trauma, will be reflected in our nervous system and the way it functions in response. The *I can* (move through this situation) version of trauma codes are created and perpetuated in our sympathetic nervous system's fight, flight, and **fawn** responses, while the *I can't* (move through this situation) version of trauma codes are created and perpetuated in our dorsal vagal parasympathetic nervous system's freeze response. A state of presence and the ability to process through our experiences is a function of the ventral vagal parasympathetic nervous system (rest and digest).[4] When we are in a state of fear, our body's nervous system is simultaneously sending us into a state of fight, flight, or fawn, and if we are unable to move out of the dynamic using these strategies our state of arousal will increase, and we will move into a state of freeze or collapse. As each of us is unique, we'll usually have a predisposition to express one type of response more than another, while the **stacking** of different responses

4   Stephen W. Porges, *The Polyvagal Theory: Neurophysiological Foundations of Emotions, Attachment, Communication, and Self-regulation.* New York: W.W. Norton, 2011.

is also common as we continue to run the same programs throughout our lives.

When we are in fear, we are unable to process our thoughts and emotions at the moment because our earthsuit is prioritizing more important functions (like a faster heartbeat in order to promote agility, or releasing glucose for quick energy). For example, we need energy to run away from danger (flight), or to fight a jaguar or tiger attack (fight). In an attack like 9/11, we may go into a state of complete shock to protect our psyche (freeze). The activation of our sympathetic nervous system can also be covert, for example if our attacker (mental, emotional, physical, or spiritual) is also a loved one, we may learn to do what is needed of us to avoid aggression (fawn). As children, we can feel unsafe in a family dynamic or in a school environment much more than you would think, and for the simple reason that we aren't offered enough presence to learn to be with the full spectrum of life as we grow. States of fear are embedded into the fabric of our current landscape, and they can be emotional, mental, spiritual, as well as physical; all will affect our well-being.

From the vantage point of the nervous system, it's our ventral vagal parasympathetic nervous system response that creates a state of safety in our human experience. In this state we trust life, our heart beats slower, and we learn to respond rather than react. It's here where we digest our food, feel our emotions, connect with others in a healthy and co-creative way, and where our bodies can regenerate and heal. An embodied knowing of our inner truth is fostered in the parasympathetic nervous system response because when our being deems the outside world safe, we can then comfortably focus our energy on our own selves. There is also good news because we can re-teach our bodies to rest in the ventral vagal parasympathetic nervous system at any age, and there are many techniques and modalities that have already been created to help us do this. As children, the spectrum of life that we experience in the state of rest and digest will mirror what was given to us from our caregivers, and the bigger the bandwidth we receive, the more our soul-self can integrate into our experience as we grow. If we weren't offered a large emotional bandwidth in presence as children, we can always expand our **window of tolerance**[5] later on through inner work.

***

There are many generational and societal programs that don't support the growth of trauma-free programming in our children, and yet they are so embedded in our culture that we don't always see them. For example, we say "It's just in the movies," but that's not really true because entertainment is our programming, and what we watch programs our aura, *especially* as children.

Let's do a little experiment. I'd like to invite you to go back to your divine inner child for a moment and ask yourself what would be the most traumatic situations for that divine inner child to witness? Did having one of your parents die make the top of the list? Well, have you ever noticed how many mothers die or are already dead in Disney movies? A few that I grew up with are *Aladdin*, *Bambi*, *Cinderella*, *Beauty and the Beast*, *Sleeping Beauty*, and *The Lion King* (where the father dies). You could argue that's just how the world is, that light and dark are a part of life, and that that's what makes a good movie. However, at this time in our history, evidence is available to suggest that these narratives were placed in our early

5   Daniel J. Siegel, *Mindsight: The New Science of Personal Transformation*. New York: Brilliance Publishing, 2015.

childhood classics as a way to create unconscious trauma for the purpose of control. In our collective reality as we live it now, we accept heartbreaking experiences as a normal part of our template, but to the human soul according to natural law—we should rightfully be given the choice. Considering that children are pure, it may be important to know who is creating our programming and their agenda. At the very minimum, knowledge propels transformation, and as a collective if we can create healthier and trauma-free content for the youngest members of the human race, why wouldn't we?

Chapter Eleven: After We Open the Door to Healing, Sometimes the Pain Comes

Do you remember the story I told you about the red dress with the blue leaves and feeling like a million bucks? I felt like this because in a moment of grace, the door to my heart opened, and I was able to remember who I was at a soul level. In the excitement of this reunion, I experienced a partial unfreezing of Soldier Al, and it wasn't until a week later that I was able to feel into the pain which was also there. My vantage point had migrated, and the ease and brightness I felt when my heart first opened was replaced by a level of emotional pain that felt worse than ever before. Just like the birds and the trees that now felt beautifully alive, I could also feel the pain of life so deeply, while before I only knew my own story. I was discovering that my heart, in its opening toward the goodness of my soul, had become more tender in its expression.

Fortunately, there was a difference this time. Another part of my vantage point had changed as well, and I now understood that I was not the pain, while in the past I had identified with it. A new piece of my consciousness had awoken, which knew that my emotions and thoughts were changeable pieces of the whole. Now that my soul was making itself known, I had a strong internal compass guiding me to move toward the higher vibrational truths of who I really was. My newly awoken soul let me know which parts of my physiology, psychology, emotionality, and life goals were no longer in alignment with who my soul was wanting me to become. The life I used to know that propelled me forward in the world (or outer being) suddenly stopped, and my focus became aimed toward the deeper parts of my foundations. I became interested in my family lineage, and letting go of any harmful acts I was still taking part in. The process this initiated allowed me to step outside myself to see the programs I was running without judgment. I also discovered that the further I could step away from myself, the deeper I could go within and claim the things I was disconnected from with compassion. I was learning how to hold the pain in the palm of my hand, and then how to place it lovingly into my heart.

After my heart first opened, I quickly decided I needed a teacher. So, I did the most rational thing I could think of . . . I opened my computer, clicked into Google, and typed "spiritual teacher, Ottawa." The first person to appear in my search was a woman wearing white. Like Snatam Kaur she was smiling and glowing back at me, so I decided to email her. "I have been away traveling," she explained in her reply a month later, and "Yes, you can book an appointment with me." When I wrote to her I was feeling bliss, but by the time we were able to meet a month later, I was feeling some deep and intense pain. I walked in for my appointment and instantly felt magic. Tucked away on a quiet street, it was a colorful space of swirling artwork, where cooking spice and incense filled the air. I immediately felt cared for. The woman who was waiting inside showed me to my seat, answered all of my questions, and mentioned the existence of aliens. I then immediately began to feel like it was my time to leave. Something was telling me from somewhere beyond, that this interaction was getting too lit up; both at a physical capacity in my cells, as well as intuitively through the light of awareness into seeing too much of my shadow.

My social skills were much less refined at that time, so my spontaneous tactic was to worm myself lower and lower in the chair where I was sitting until finally, I could slink myself away. The tactic was successful, but not quickly enough. Before I could make my move, she spoke a phrase that cracked me open yet again. She told me I was a healer. I responded, bewildered and defensive, "No, I'm going to be an architect." What she said scared me deeply because it required me to give up my entire life plan. *Great*, I thought, *like I need even more reasons to feel like my world is crumbling at my feet!*

***

I was not a child who was capable of integrating the full spectrum of my emotional world through the support of the adults who were available to me in early life. Instead, Soldier Al continued to do his work of freezing out the pain near my heart until much later on in my journey. Plus, to make matters slightly worse, in this type of situation (one where we haven't yet learned the power of presence), the original trauma will continue to get stacked up with new experiences, which are running on the same foundations. There are two vantage points that I find helpful when explaining why this happens. The first, is to understand that trauma is an unconscious and incomplete energetic charge that is propelling itself forward in a desire to be completed. This happens because our natural desire for presence is always moving us towards wholeness (even if that movement is unconscious to us). The second is to see it exactly as it is, a program that is coded as incomplete, which means there is a stuck emotion. The crossroads between these two vantage points is what keeps us recreating our woes and reliving the same joys. Many of us have lived unconscious to the codes that we carry, and because of it we've been able to accumulate quite a pile of experiences.

That's why awakening spiritually is often birthed out of a place of pain. It is when we are at our lowest of lows, when the weight of life becomes unbearable, that we cry out to more than ourselves, and for another way. When we exercise our free will in this way—with a desire to break out of the places we find ourselves, grace can arrive, extend its hand, and offer us a taste of something more. When this happens, life is never the same again. For me, after my unexpected moment in heaven, it was like God had decided to take the cross from the top of the steeple and bring it down only for me. He had heard me cry, and so he said, "Okay my dear, I see that you've had enough of how you've been . . . so, are you ready to take responsibility for your actions in a very real way? Are you ready to live a life of ownership and sovereignty? Are you ready to take your power back?" In my bravery I said yes, and then a new journey began.

There are many symbolic interpretations of the cross and when this big shift took place for me, I experienced some of these interpretations. In my worst moments, when the emotional and psychological pain would get too strong, it felt like I was attending my own crucifixion. Then, as I found ways to transmute the pain I was holding on to, I also experienced the cross as the horizontal and vertical planes of the human expression. The cross' vertical axis meant spending time in my central channel doing inner work, and its horizontal axis meant my expression of that inner alchemy as I naturally shared my gifts and learnings with others. Notably, the place where these two worlds meet (internal and external) is the heart. As I learned through experience, one constant remained: I was asked to become responsible for my actions to the degree that it would become a lifelong investigation into learning to master my life force.

My next seven years were spent studying inside the expansive world of the healing arts. I explored spirituality, yoga, meditation, shamanism, plant medicine, and energy healing (all of which I am a lifelong student). Since then, in my time spent working with my own pain and the pain of others, this has become my list of tips to support the process:

Tips for finding, holding, and processing your pain.

1. All the ways that you feel called to heal will be the right ways for you. No one person's journey is the same, so don't worry about doing things the right or wrong way. What's most important is that you let your inner compass guide you.

2. Accept and fall in love with your shadow. We all have one, and a lot of life force can be wasted in judgment or through pretending that it doesn't exist.

3. When you are healing a specific belief or emotion, it can feel as if that emotion or belief has complete control over you. Sometimes it does. But if you stay connected to your light, (which is first portrayed through the archetype of your divine inner child), the moment you are able to surrender yourself from the depths is the moment that God's grace can step in and take away your inner battle for you. Sometimes, we battle for what seems like eternity, yet the process has been initiated because we are meant to learn something. Find that thing. Shine a flashlight on it, and with humility, you can then let God take over.

4. Sometimes the mechanics of your nervous system (moving from fear to love) seem unchangeable and beyond your control; in these situations remember

that compassion is a master healer, and that shifts in the body take time.

5. Be patient with yourself.

6. Take a daily dose of self-forgiveness, and practice forgiving others.

7. Invite your inner warrior to step in and show you how certain they are that you can do this.

This chapter speaks to what might happen to you if your beautiful soul chooses to open up your heart in the middle of your life, and the pain that you may have to work through when it does. To better understand the type of inner program that you might find yourself reading, I'm going to bring back the example of the little boy who had his toy taken away from him (enough times to create a pattern), when he was only two—except now he is thirty-eight. In this scenario, just like I was at twenty-four, Jim has not yet become aware of the foundational programs he has which hold pain, and now that he's an adult, here are some ways that this same program could continue to reappear. Like Soldier Al, I've given his program a name. Consider it as an early relational trauma,[1] that can be associated with not only toys, but with other living beings too.

The Energetic Program of No Boundaries Bob.

Subtle Sensations: A sensation of being punched in the stomach when something is taken from him, and then a numbness that engulfs him.

---

1   John Bowlby, _A Secure Base: Parent-Child Attachment and Healthy Human Development_. London: Routledge, 1988.

Instinctual Emotions: A feeling of fear that arises spontaneously when he is close to someone/something he loves or cares for deeply. A feeling of deep sadness when he no longer has what he loves.

Beliefs: A silhouetted figure who shows up out of the blue to take away something that belongs to him. The unconscious belief Bob creates is, "Things I enjoy can and will be taken away from me without warning and without my consent, I must not be worthy of love."

Relational Emotions and Soul Lessons: This man's soul lesson is to learn through the experience of having the things he loves taken away from him without his consent. His soul is propelling him towards the discovery that he deserves to love and be loved, in a safe and non-threatening way.

Trauma-Free Template: Once this man learns that healthy boundaries are a part of his basic needs, he will be able to give and receive love more fluidly, more easefully, and with more fulfillment and stability. Perhaps he will also be able to surrender when things are taken from him or someone leaves outside his control.

The programming that Jim carries, unconsciously instructs him to stay away from his pain, and the type of sympathetic nervous system response his being will choose in order to keep this program running will depend on his disposition, while cycling through different responses at different times is also common. Here is an example of how all four sympathetic nervous system responses could manifest later on in Jim's life:

Fight Response: He creates a position of power where he can have more control over his reality and when his relationships or belongings feel threatened, he becomes aggressive.

Flight Response: He develops a resistance to owning material things or experiencing intimate relationships.

Freeze Response: He experiences a series of relationships that end abruptly and unexpected, leaving him paralyzed and confused.

Fawn Response: He gives his time and belongings away to others in a way that depletes his cup rather than overflows it. He has more control over his pain if he is the one who manages it.

When I support others in the process of opening up to the vibration of their divine inner child, something else commonly happens. Other parts of their inner child also show up: the wounded parts. It's the parts of them who were left home alone, or fell off their bike, or much worse than that. The voice of these parts is human trauma in whatever capacity it was created, and then a couple of different things usually happen next. The first is that it becomes easier for that person to have compassion for themselves, as they can now see the innocent foundations behind some of their coping strategies. Many people instantly turn from self-judgment to tears, and that's a lovely heart-opening moment. The second thing is that those people who think that they can move through the healing process using sheer force of will, realize that they're going to have to slow down and take a different approach. These people then learn how to focus their efforts on building a bridge of trust between the aspects of themselves that feel unsafe or unseen, and the safe parts of themselves that are living in the present moment. It becomes a process of learning patience, of learning to release control, and of learning to love themselves just as they are while still aspiring to become who they want to be.

When we experience things as children from the world around us that are negative or unsafe, and there is no one there to help us process through it, we think that we're responsible, which is how that experience becomes internalized as an unconscious program. We will think we're responsible because we don't yet have a fully developed ego. Our biofield is still growing, and so we naturally acknowledge the other as us. It is also a survival tactic because from the perspective of a child, it's safer to think that we are at fault, than accept the truth of our reality as being unsafe around us. In the moment of the program's creation it's a life-preserving choice made by our earth-suit as we integrate into the matrix, however, if these childhood responses never get updated we'll continue to live in the same self-preserving childish way when triggered. This is the part of us who holds us back, gets jealous, is controlling, is afraid of intimacy, is too needy, still has a temper tantrum, and has internalized negative self-talk. They are the parts of us that need our attention because they are holding us back from expressing the fullness of who we truly are. These are the parts of our inner gardens that now need our love.

***

Deep soul healing is at times painful (there is no way around it). Through the eyes of your divine inner child, any trespass you have experienced will need to pass through your heart in order for it to be absolved. A soul-based perspective also shows us that anything that is an affront to our soul, is also a trespass we have done to ourselves. For example, if we are the aggressor in our current experience, in another life we were the victim. **Karma** is a balancing of the scales, meaning that any actions we have taken in other lives will likely be recreated and done to us in a future life. It's not punishment, it's the balancing of the cosmic inhale and exhale. We also have the birthright to go within and to release ourselves from its bondage. In truth, we are not separate from anything, but the experience of polarity makes us see that we are only one side of the coin. To move through karma in this life, balance through lesson learning is what brings our painful experiences through the eye of the needle or in this case, through the portal in the heart. When we become both sides of our dilemma through inner work, we can reconcile differences, understand, see, learn, forgive ourselves, and set a future self view. In doing so, we complete the lesson, absolve the program through heart magic, and then in time, we can move forward towards our next adventure with more space in our being to do so.

Chapter Twelve:
The Spirit of Religion and Navigating Relationships

The backyard studio where my heart first opened to the remembrance of my soul, abutted a two-story, red brick Italian wartime house where I lived alongside four housemates during my time as an architecture student. People came and went: fellow architects in training, transient exchange students, and a sprinkle of students from other degrees just to spice things up. We had style—it was the party house.

The spring before I went to university, my father decided it would be a good investment to buy a house and to rent its rooms to other students as I completed my studies. It was a new venture that had us house hunting all summer long; we looked in the suburbs, at a house with a pool, and then we landed at 99 Young Street, a small wartime home turned convent for a group of Catholic nuns who belonged to the church across the street. They ran a tight and organized ship. The house was kept in order with masking tape labels and the creative installation of walls made from curtains—which gave a whole new meaning to the term curtain wall, and turned a home built for five into seven. My move to 99 Young Street was prior to learning that I could read energy, and looking back, I must have been subconsciously attracted to the clarity that a space devoted to God had created.

What are your thoughts on God and religion? Yes, I just threw that enormous question at you with little warning. But it's here now, written, frozen in time as words on a page, so welcome to the conversation! Take a moment and allow your perspective to stay true in your own heart. Breathe and take a pause. If you are religious in any way, take a moment to connect to your faith. Notice if it feels true in your core and if it gives positive meaning to your life. If that's the way you feel, keep that feeling close and stay curious for this next bit. If religion is a sensitive and personal subject for you, you could consider gently skipping this chapter, while if you are someone who feels uncertain or resistant to religion, the following perspective might be insightful, as it has been influenced by my understanding of how our consciousness develops as children. I am choosing to shed light on this subject because, sometimes when we are raised in a religion, its indoctrination can create a program that inhibits our soul from living its fullness through our human body.

Now, before I begin to deconstruct an institution that many people would consider sacred, I'd like you to know that I have much respect for the desire to do good, and affinity to a higher power that calls people to a faith. I love Jesus and his teachings and still do today, but for someone who believes that we co-create our realities anew in every moment, I do consider the narrative I was offered through the religion I was raised in to be an incomplete one. Meaning that it is missing some important teachings, which, I believe, were removed over time. That's because my experience never pointed me toward myself in the deeper way that I needed. My experience with religion was missing the feminine principles, or in other words, it was missing the teachings of embodiment.

I was raised in the Catholic faith. I went to Catholic school from kindergarten until grade twelve; I wore uniforms and I learned that Jesus was the only son of God. Since before I can remember, I learned to recite certain prayers and creeds, and the story of Jesus in the way he was presented by the Catholic Church was told to me as an absolute truth. Along with all the memorizing and reciting that was going on in my childhood, from a familial level, I also have many good memories too. Snippets of family phrases that I remember with a sense of endearment. They were full of authority and anchored in silliness, as they bellowed through my family's house on Sunday mornings as a kid. "Hurry up, I'm waiting in the car! . . . Jesus, Mary, and Joseph we are going to be late!" . . . and "don't wear jeans!"

In my more recent years, I began researching the origins of the Catholic Church when a past life memory of mine came forward. While in training to become a yoga teacher, a seasoned healer came in one day and graced us with her presence. She led us through a shamanic journey and as the drum beat, we sank deeper and deeper into our personal depths. That's when a vision came through me of a lifetime I had spent as a high authority in the church. It was quite revealing. Tall and slim, and adorned in robes, I witnessed myself playing a role as a bad character in the church's inner circle. A piece of information I hope society will soon embrace is that at the very top of our systems (not just in the church) there is actually an inversion of intent, and this is why we continue to experience pain and suffering.

Pain and suffering are not expressions that are inherent in human beings, but a collectively chosen program. In my past life memory as a high-ranking priest, and conscious of how the energy bodies functioned, I understood that if the human **dantian point** was compromised at a young age, people could be more easily controlled. The creation of a religious system that is heavy with indoctrination is not a fluke, and from what I have learned thus far, the Catholic Church did not start out so disconnected from the teachings of the soul. Instead, this separation evolved over time, and especially after the Council of Nicea in 325 AD. It was around this time that the masculine principles, which supported a more structural understanding of right and wrong, dominated and eventually deleted the gnostic or feminine principles of introspection and soul sovereignty from their teachings.[1] If the masculine is the structure (something that the Catholic Church does well), then the feminine is that which fills it (something which is better offered in the yogic traditions).[2]

My past life memory stirred my curiosity, and I now understand that the system I was raised in taught me to take the essence of Christ consciousness in from the external environment, rather than a system that taught me to nurture that same Christ consciousness from the inside out through soul sovereignty. If you are someone who believes that humans are the collective creators of their reality, then it means that as soon as we change a personal or collective belief, that our reality will change too. In the creed of my religion, I was taught that Jesus was crucified, and that he did so to take away our sins. Perhaps this is true, yet as I began to shed my indoctrinations' pinpointed focus, I've become acquainted with new and lighter beliefs that have taught me how to learn from and heal my own sins. These are the same beliefs that I am sharing with you in this book.

------

1   Tricia McCannon, *Return of the Divine Sophia: Healing the Earth Through the Lost Wisdom Teachings of Jesus, Isis and Mary Magdalene* (Vermont: Bear & Company, 2015), 245-389.

2   Paranhamsa Yogananda, *The Essence of the Bhagavad Gita, Explained by Paranhamsa Yogananda, As Remembered by His Disciple, Swami Kriyananda*. Nevada City: Crystal Clarity Publishers, 2006.

The older I grew, and without knowing any of the factual details until much later, I naturally began to feel that the Catholic way of thinking didn't sit right with me. Yet, since these beliefs were taught to me as the absolutes, they were tough ones for me to dislodge from my sense of self. That's probably why I became an atheist for a time, as dropping all faith in anything allowed those old, indoctrinated beliefs to loosen their energetic stronghold. You've now learned that from a subtle energetic perspective that's really what they are . . . beliefs attached to a strong emotion and anchored into place through a sensation in the body. When they are given to us as children, before our full sense of individuation has been fostered, they become a part of our reality's foundation.

Have you ever been in the forest or gone for a walk in the city and seen a tree that's grown around a rock, a fence, or some sort of man-made object? If you haven't, I suggest you Google it. Being indoctrinated is like being the tree that's grown around a fence or rock, and in the process, the tree (you) and the object (indoctrination) have become integral in each other's experience. Where a larger tree would easily knock the fence over, children are like the little sapling learning to grow on a forest trail. For an older tree, who's already grown around the fence, it may need that fence to stay in place for good health, while for another tree the fence may be six feet away, and so it doesn't interfere with its core boundaries.

The rigidity of beliefs, which can also be seen as structural support, are an innate aspect of human nature, and a vital component of a healthy, happy, and purpose-filled life. Think about what it would be like to have no bones to give us shape, no skin to hold in our vital organs, and no job or loved ones to give our lives a sense of purpose. We need structure to function. Humans are a matrix of the form and formless, the yin and yang, the known and the unknown, and the list goes on! What doesn't work is, if those particular structures or beliefs are not a vibrational match to our own unique soul tone and psychic being. If the beliefs you have adopted as a child are too far away from how you want to express your unique individuation as an adult, things will feel off.

At the same time, this process of adopting beliefs is natural as we grow up. It creates the foundations for our next stage of development, when we come to know our unique purpose through our individuation. So, if our set of given beliefs offer us this capacity to know our purpose, then they will work, and if they don't, they will feel wrong to us. Our brain fully develops around the age of twenty-five,[3] and it's my belief that before this age, we are in service to our unconscious programs because we can not yet fully self-reflect. It's also during and after this age that we may need to shed and adopt new beliefs and habits, once we grow to become capable of doing so.

From the heart's perspective, we are equal and unique, and just like the brilliance of nature from which we are not separate, an open heart emits a resonance that says that we all have a reason for being alive that supports the greatness of the whole. We are diverse, and so it's not about if religion is right or wrong, it's about if your relationship to it fosters a sense of purpose and individuation of belonging for you. I am a lover of beauty myself—I consider it a part of the highest order, and I know that there is grace and brilliance laced in lineages of faith and the rituals behind them. I consider their many unique tones of sacred heritage important, and when we choose to travel the road within, many of those roads are steeped in religion's

3   "Brain Maturity Extends Well Beyond Teen Years," NPR (website), last updated October 10, 2011, https://www.npr.org/templates/story/story.php?storyId=141164708

sacred knowledge too. The key factor is that our faith is something we feel a kinship with, which allows us to feel more connected to our sense of purpose, community, and safety in our existence as a human being. Your faith has to be in alignment with whom you truly are, and only you can decide that.

***

In Richard Rudd's book *The Gene Keys*, he says that genius is "the innate intelligence of all human beings," and that "true genius is a spontaneous and creative uniqueness rooted in unconditional love. Genius is the natural manifestation of a human life when it is allowed to expand without force."[4] This is done when we support the growth of our emotional energy and practice using the power of our subtle heart by allowing our natural-ness to question and *try on for size* the beliefs that we are given from the outside world. We are swapping out authority and control, for self-reflection and freedom of expression. When we support this model in our children, we are allowing them to expand their capacity to self-reg-ulate and be present by allowing them to honor, feel, and process their innate emotional responses. Richard Rudd's model corresponds to a healthy dantian point, which is the area of our energetic anatomy that directs the power of our personal life force.

***

In this new paradigm or thought, it's an accepted truth that the human species is an interconnected web of light; that there is no such thing as separation. We often learn this when our soul activates, and becoming conscious to it is like waking up from one version of a dream and

---

4   Richard Rudd, *Gene Keys: Unlocking the Higher Purpose Hidden in Your DNA* (London: Watkins, 2015), 525.

walking into another. When this happens we may choose to make changes to the vibration of our reality, and if we do, this choice will also mean re-patterning the frequency of those connections that are closest to us. In this case, since we are the ones who are choosing to change, we are also given the responsibility of navigating the bulk of the evolving connections within our families and close friends.

Imagine this: every one of us is a pole in a massive party tent that covers the entire planet. When we are a part of the current paradigm's matrix of life, we are standing tall in the **third density**: the dimension of personal will and power, and a dimension governed by our solar plexus. Let's say that these tent people are ten feet tall (an arbitrary height that has no correlation to hierarchy). Those of us who feel called to evolve into more of our souls' nature will go through a process of having our tent pole rise higher into the **fourth density** (into heart-centered consciousness), and eventually into the **fifth density** (into soul sovereignty). Let's say that these tent people are about fifteen feet tall. As we evolve, relational issues arise because the party tent is covered in fabric, and that fabric is connected to the tent poles beside it.

Our family members and long-term relationships are the poles closest to us and when we make changes to ourselves, we will also be affecting them. Inevitably there will be tension, and until both people are able to express their new boundaries, a tug of war is created between the evolving tent person and the tent people closest to them. The dynamics of this shift can be seen through the evolving tent person's natural need to be approved by those who they are closest to, or through the disregard for those same people's needs (resistance will manifest through polarities). Our neighboring tent people may also create tension because humans aren't too keen when it comes to accepting change that they didn't choose themselves.

What I've found to be a good rule of thumb, is to notice that keeping your own cup overflowing through the process is different from pouring your cup into other people's cups. When I've overstepped my boundaries or depleted myself supporting another in an unbalanced way, I take a step back and put my trust in a universe that is working for the best possible outcome for all beings. Ultimately, it is a game of knowing that we can recreate new boundaries through love, and that the only person we can truly change is ourselves. When you are in the process of raising your frequency into the fourth density (the density of healing separation) and eventually into the fifth, handiwork is required to be done on the fabric between tent poles, to allow both parties to stand at a height where they feel comfortable. There is no way around this process, and the fabric's retrofitting will happen in a way that's unique to each of us. The path you walk to get there will be your own, and I hope my list of tips helps to support you in doing just that.

Tips for navigating heart-centered relationship transitions:

1. Love other people in the same way you would like to be loved, or even better, in the way they would like to be loved.
2. Share your truth and listen to other people's truths.
3. Ask questions if you don't know the answers.
4. Hold space for loving dialogue.
5. Acknowledge your own needs, and the needs of others.
6. Give others the opportunity and responsibility to know and share their needs.

7. Envision the best possible outcome for your situation, then hold it clear yet without attachment.

8. Sometimes unwanted outcomes are the true outcomes and if these come to pass, a continual eminence of unconditional love from afar leaves the door open for more transformation in the future.

9. If your family and close friends are unable to support the changes you want to make to your personal boundaries, find a safe group of people (a class or a support group) to **hold space** for your transition. Sometimes we are even strong enough to make these changes on our own through meditation, breathwork, and a connection to our higher self or to God.

10. Stay close to your divine inner child.

11. Stay close to gratitude.

12. The best possible outcome is to keep our loved ones close while transforming our relational dynamics with them, yet know that if they are unable to make these changes with you, that a new person will come in to take their place in due time. There is pain in loss, but it's only to make space for more light in your experience over time.

At the beginning of awakening to your soul, your experiences can seem as though your family is the culprit for many of the problems you experience as you learn to integrate the pain you have lived separated from. But go easy on them and think of it more like you are moving out of the current collective issues that affect all of humanity, and try to honor both experiences as valuable in the grand scheme of things. Remember how I told you that the biggest field wins? Oftentimes, when we first awaken, it will be our families' field that wins. So, it's a good idea to find an additional safe space for yourself in those early moments of change. After that, my advice is to make your changes slowly and intentionally, allowing those around you space for their own comfort and necessary adjustments. Sometimes though, like the forest fire that causes devastating, drastic, and immediate change, or a bridge that breaks in the wake of a tsunami, things can happen in an instant. But like the slower decomposition of an old wooden barn along the rainy roadside of a forested small town, it can also happen over a long period of time, and if we can foresee the shift and do it slowly, there is less room for trauma. That is the flow of change that I aim for, and all of these ways are natural to earth as we ride the wave of evolution.

Within your subtle anatomy, much like the fabric of the tent that connects the tent poles, you have heart strings (sometimes considered heart ropes), that form to connect your relationships with other beings. If someone exists in your reality, even for just a conversation, there will be subtle lines of energy that connect you to them (chakra to chakra), and the more time you spend together, the stronger those lines will become. These lines of energy don't just connect to the heart, as **relational cords** can be created through any of your chakras, which are created depending on what parts of your expression you are relating with the most.

In the mainstream matrix, a majority of these lines of energy will be connected in a third density way, which means that their mode of operation will be firstly through control (mostly unconscious) as the third chakra is all about power. In third density relating, once the boundaries of that relationship have been established, then love will grow within that structure, while when we shift into the heart, unconditional love has the opportunity to become our foundation. The power dynamics and rigidity of the boundaries we created in that relationship then play a secondary role. Sometimes when we start changing our foundational programs, the relationships that were anchored in our old beliefs don't make it through the shifts, and we wonder why the love seems to have disappeared into thin air. It's why unconditional love and heart-centered relationships, where we see the soul of another, can also dissolve old relational boundaries and create new ones as we make adjustments to our own.

It's not our place to change others. Yet because our early relational programs are based on how we've responded to our parents and closest caregivers, or how they have responded to us, the programs that will need changing usually become activated and apparent when we are relating to them or to our own families through this new lens. When and if this happens to you, instead of bringing forth issues from the past to be hashed out unannounced (which is how those who are involved may interpret it), try this: an energetic technique that pulls your relational cords back toward yourself so that you can become both sides of the dynamic.

An Energetic Technique to Dissolve Old Relational Cords:

In your inner world (perhaps with the support of a guided meditation), you can imagine playing out both parts of the scenario at hand. Ownership in this way creates an internal reconciliation dynamic, and with your inner vision, you can then ask the hurt parts of you what they need, and aim to meet those needs. It's a technique that takes any blame or stuckness that you may carry within, and reorients it toward the energy of transformation. Unless the person on the other end of your relational cords is capable of a heart-centered conversation, the changes you are desiring to create may not be possible for them to comprehend. Remember that you are the one asking to be in a relationship with your divine inner child, and to strengthen that relationship you may need to acknowledge and honor their needs in the areas where your parents were not able to in the past. You become your own parent, the one you needed but didn't have. Meeting your own basic needs in this way (organically and over time), will create healthier foundational templates within, and once you've managed that, you'll be propelled to create new relational cords with others in the now. With your growing level of personal power, these new relational cords will then become a reflection of the wholeness that you've already created within.

The time has come for your next assignment, but first, please take a breath. Notice your face, is it smiling or serious . . . contented or confused. Check in with yourself and take another breath all the way down to your toes. Your next assignment is to take a moment and see if you can find any parallels from what you've just learned in your life (in the ways that society functions), to the dynamics that have been established in your family. Notice what parts of you are relating from the heart and what parts of you are relating through power (or powerlessness). These dynamics can be covert, but all of us will have them because we are all human. These are the dynamics currently imbued into our collective fabric, and the dynamics that will need your attention.

***

When you grow into your light, you can inadvertently trigger others with your brightness. That's because their demons (or unconscious pain) may use a tactic of projecting the things that are holding them back from their light, out and into their field so that their auric screen reads the external environment as being those same demons. It might make them run from you, shut down, or perceive you as the enemy. On the other hand, if they trust you and are willing to take in the new information you are emanating, I've noticed that it can make people fall asleep.

For example, in the wake of writing this book, I excitedly gave my friend a ten-minute explanation of the work I was doing. Her response was, "Wow, that was a lot of information, Marnie. I am going to take a nap now." We were sitting in the back seat of my father's truck driving to visit my grandfather, and she immediately proceeded to take a ten-minute nap, seemingly out of the blue. I overloaded her, and I learned again the importance of baby steps. When we shift paradigms both in ourselves and in our relationships, it's important to remember that the body has to physically evolve in order to take in new levels of light, and even if both parties hold positivity for the process, it's something that inherently takes time and patience.

Chapter Thirteen:
Soldier Al
In The Flesh

In the healing arts, it's commonly accepted that trauma gets passed down in family lines for seven generations. So inevitably, healing ourselves in a deeper way will include healing those parts of our lineage that still hold pain. For example, if your grandfather or great-grandfather experienced a world war and never went through a healing process for what they experienced, you could be holding an evolution of their trauma in your own energy field today (and also their fabulous courage). The restrictions to presence that trauma creates gets passed down through family lines, and once the trauma's expression is removed from its original context, the symptoms we see can appear through addiction, dysfunctional habits, or as subtleties in our personality. The subtleties of generational pain hold us back from expressing our best selves because they also restrict our gifts, and we will pass those same tendencies on to our own children as they grow up if we don't wake up to what we're carrying. When it comes to generational pain, if we are conscious, capable, and feel the call, it's my opinion that we have a sacred duty to process and acknowledge that pain which activates the courage which is also encoded. Just like inheritance comes with as many musty old sweaters as it does jewels to be enjoyed, some heart-centered spring cleaning every once in a generation is required to keep our lineage healthy and flourishing.

I have met many sensitive and gifted humans who became overwhelmed by the pain of humanity that they decided to live off the grid away from the matrix. Even if you aren't one of these people, there is medicine in noticing that we are in pain as a collective. In the mainstream matrix we have become quite disconnected from the pain (and also the innate joy) that we carry, and so we continue to manifest the pain outwards through unconscious action, not seeing a connection between its different layers of expression. We have lived on the surface of things, while for many of us that truth is now changing.

States of balance and harmony within us will manifest into the world as such, and the same goes for states of pain. My intention is not to go all *dark side* on you, but I do feel this next bit must be said because for a species who from a soul-level is naturally centered in the purity of the heart, the trauma-based system that we live in is harming us; war, rape, and greed are hurting us and causing a sickness within our psyche.

If you are someone who feels as if you are not affected by any of these big themes, consider that they are also energies that live within all of us as programs. Just as world news travels, no one is excluded from knowing these because we are all a part of humanity's web. For example, when was the last time you were critical and judgmental toward yourself or others? This way of living carries the same seed as war. When was the last time you ate or bought something without pausing to acknowledge where it came from, who cared for or created it, and what mother earth had to give forth in order for it to exist? This way of living carries the same seed as rape. When was the last time you took more than you needed, or filled your own cup to the point of overflowing without feeling the need to share that flow with others? This way of living carries the same seed as greed. Yes, they are much more subtle in their expressions, but they have the same root, and by bringing this truth to light through curiosity and love, we learn first hand that we cannot judge another without first judging ourselves. Plus if we are devoted enough to our efforts as a collective, we also have the ability to let go of the energies of rape, war, and greed completely.

Change within equals change without, and since we all hold the codes of humanity we are all responsible for making these changes, by first changing our own programs.

***

As we walk the path of the soul, we are inviting more and more light to enter our physical body, which translates to more personal power as we co-create with life. We are choosing to turn up our personal power and what we think and feel—good and bad—will begin to manifest more quickly. The part of us that is conscious, however, is not wholly in charge of this process because the conscious part of us is just the tip of the manifesting iceberg. We are also manifesting from the rest of the iceberg that is holding its position in the depths of the ocean. That's why taking a scuba dive with our conscious mind from time to time allows us to discover why we are manifesting the things that we don't actually want in our lives.

Consciously choosing what you'd like to manifest can be a fun and empowering energetic tool that you may have heard of, but in my case it was not a fun *manifest your dreams* sort of manifesting project. The dreams of joy I had in mind still needed to have work done to their foundations. Instead my current project went something like this: *I want to build my life in this old house, but some of its inheritance is smelling very musty, I think it's time to do some spring cleaning and I really don't know what I am going to find, so best I wear the rubber gloves* type of conscious manifesting. Instead of watching TV or choosing to talk to a friend, I chose to walk into the unknown territory of my inner landscape. As spiritual lingo would have it, I wanted to get to know the next layer of the onion and unbeknownst to me until it happened, my time spent in meditation created a strong and obvious reflection in my waking world. A reflection expressed through the arrival of Al the roommate: a tall, brown-haired, hazel-eyed viking and real-life physical human.

The months I spent with Al did not go down as my favorite months of the year. I'd like to say he arrived like a knight in shining armor as I began to unfreeze the dormant energies within me, but that was not the case. My viking soldier arrived traumatized and severely distrusting of everything in his surroundings (in the way someone unfreezing from holding a lifetime of pain probably would). Al arrived ill and his lack of energy made it hard to see his underlying power. I knew Al the roommate before he came to live with me, and it's why I spontaneously let him move in. Although not native to the land, I had met Al as a young man in India and now nine years later he was looking for a temporary place to stay in Vancouver. It was easy for me to crush on the star-like qualities that I had remembered him to embody, but my initial fantasies quietly faded, as I realized that this person was much different than I had remembered him to be. What started off as a kind friendship inspired by the intention to support each other's professional growth, soon took a turn for the worse as the shadows of my own relational programming began to reveal themselves, and with them my heart began to feel battered and numb.

The certain goodness that I first felt about Al's essence, was getting sidelined as his presence triggered fears I didn't even know that I carried, and they came fourth from my heritage and collective disempowerment of the feminine. In its broadest archetypal form, it's through our inability to *be* as a collective, which is the essence of the feminine, that we have created opportunities for all sorts of painful programs to stay running rampant in our experience. Instead, we zoom past the pain and ignore the delicate disposition that femininity needs in order to bloom.

In my own world, the waking up of this powerful, yet traumatized soldier got me thinking. With Al's presence in human form, my lineage patterns came to the forefront, and they were activating and unraveling quickly, like the way a movie film does as you spin it around its axis.

On the one hand, my relationship with Al was uprooting a line of playing small that was painful to see and feel, while the gift on the other hand was that I was standing in more of my power. I was now capable of staying present through my **triggers**, and that made all the difference. In my earnest desire to evolve through the relational programming that Soldier Al had been protecting my heart from, the universe had sent me a test and unlike my many romantic relationships of the past, this time I was unchained. In the experience of my pseudo partner, I was not in love and so I could see more clearly. I also had the ability to create real world boundaries through open communication, and I could choose not to invest my energy in something that did not feel like an even exchange. This time, I had become a warrior of the heart.

What is the essence of the warrior? When frozen Soldier Al unfroze, the warrior archetype awoke within me as well, surprising me with my own power. I felt angry, passionate, and fearless; a stark contrast from my usual light, loving, and non-feather-ruffling demeanour. I was full of force and I didn't know what to do with it. The thought of warriorship brought with it images of bloodshed and battlegrounds, which didn't seem right to me. Yet I was angry, and I found myself alert and learning the lethal nature of its double-edged sword; aware of the pain I could cause if ever I stopped holding that anger balanced in the palm of my hand.

In the time I spent getting to know Al the roommate, I've also opened a new file of psychic knowledge, which revealed without question the madness happening at the top echelons of our society. The False Light Matrix is what I've learned to call it, and as there is now enough transparency in our world to understand how it functions, I've been able to take a lengthy lesson in learning the depths of what Al's archetype was really protecting me from. However, the details of that file are not for this book, but I will share with you the lesson.

I learned that the warrior's truest purpose is to defend the innocent, while if I let my anger channel through me, I discovered that I could easily express violence. I was surprised. I had tapped into my rage, and once I learned where it was, I was tasked with learning how to refine its output in order to use it consciously as force. As I entered into my sacred battle, my own archetypal warrior came forth from within and with the presence of a master ninja, she was the ultimate defender of my sacred space.

Instead of blaming and fighting the external world and its demons, I became focused on removing any darkness within, whose time living in me as a program had expired. I was a warrior for my own innocence, and defending my own safe and sovereign territory was my purpose. With my soul-self activated, my inner warrior was now in service to a vaster reign of goodness and purity, which grew forth from the heart of my divine inner child.

In my interactions with Al, it became clear right away: he was living from his mind and from his power (which were both quite refined), and not from his heart. Perhaps it was because he was traumatized himself, yet it meant that every phrase of blame or guilt, every act of power that didn't first come through contemplation, and every conversation unconsciously propelled by the seeds of rape, war, and greed, were being ushered out of my relational space using the right phrase or breath from the heart. I had become strong enough to combat judgment with unconditional love.

Then in an abrupt turn of events, Al the roommate informed me one day that he would no longer be my roommate and proceeded to move out within the following hour. As it became just me again, I was left with a momentary sense of shock, and then a smile in my heart that told me that I had passed my test. On the hero's journey (just like in the movies), we'll meet allies along the way, beings from many kingdoms who come to offer their assistance, and even though Al the roommate appeared on my path as an adversary this time, from a soul level I knew we were kindred.

***

I remember an analogy from my first spiritual teacher (the one I wormed away from in my early years of awakened life) that describes the landscape of the subtle heart. It's a story, which I've embellished a little as the mind of a storyteller tends to do, and it goes like this: the inner landscape of the subtle heart is like a dinner table at Christmas. That's because to the spirit of Christmas everyone is welcome at its table, like how in the heart space everyone deserves love. Let's say that your entire family is seated around this Christmas table; aunts, uncles, cousins, mothers, fathers, grandmothers, grandfathers, close friends, babies, sisters, brothers, and all of your beloved pets. You are eating and laughing, telling stories and enjoying the celebration, but despite the joy you're experiencing, you also notice a constant knock at the door. For a while you try and ignore it because you know exactly who it is. It's Uncle Joe. He smells bad, curses a lot, and scares the children with his unfiltered version of reality. As time spent at dinner passes, the knocking doesn't cease. Instead it only gets louder and more bothersome, and to everyone seated it becomes clear that Uncle Joe is not planning to leave any time soon.

Finally, the youngest grandchild, a curly-haired, blue-eyed, three-year-old little human speaks up and says, "Why don't we let Uncle Joe inside?" Then the grandmother at the table who's been wisely watching all along, heeds the call of purity and walks over to the front door to let Uncle Joe in. At first, he yells and screams. Uncle Joe is angry, cold, and feeling abandoned, and it's true that he has caused his family a lot of pain, but that's only because he himself is in pain. Then some time passes, and over the course of the meal, Uncle Joe calms down. He is able to focus less on the pain he is in, and more on the fact that he is now enjoying his Christmas dinner. Now an aunt joins in to welcome Joe to the table, and another even apologizes for leaving him out in the cold. Uncle Joe relaxes even more.

Soul-centered love, like the spirit of Christmas dinner, offers balance and through it we can heal the pieces of us within that are constantly calling to be seen. They are the pieces of us that are knocking at the corners of our awareness, waiting at the front door of our hearts. These parts of us, who we have yet to welcome, might show up a little (or a lot) rougher around the edges, but it's only because they have been neglected. We may want to turn away from these pieces because they are not shiny and new. They may not yet function as we would like them to, and they may make us temporarily less effective in our worldly endeavors, especially when we open up to them and let them live through us as they heal. Yet the nature of love is inclusivity, and when we practice this, two things can happen next. The pieces that are us, when they truly feel seen and have their basic needs met, will settle down and unify with the whole of us. While the pieces that are not us will leave if they are unable to integrate with the coherence of our heart. Both make us more resilient and more balanced over time. Many of us think that our basic needs are food, water, and shelter, but from the moment that we are born, our baseline fundamental need is to be seen and loved in our uniqueness. It's from the building blocks of love that the world around us will naturally meet the rest of our needs.

***

I'm so glad you made it here. I've tried my best to lighten up the content of what you've just read, yet it was a deep dive even for me. You've just read through an overview of your subtle anatomy; how the layers of your energy field develops from birth and how trauma gets created in childhood; what indoctrination looks like to the energy field; how to work with and understand the energetics of your close relationships; how to relate to yourself and others from the heart and how pain may appear after you make the decision to become more connected to your soul; the importance of acknowledging generational trauma; and finally the importance of creating and knowing your own boundaries. The subject matter you've just digested was truly deep, and so I'd like to congratulate you on making it to the other side! We are now going to switch gears, and even though the content may go deeper still, it will feel lighter. Excitingly, we are near the end, and in the next chapters I'm going to share with you some of the ways I initiated vibrational healing as a balm for my own wounds by co-creating with allies from the earth.

Chapter Fourteen: The Rhodochrosite Heart

Do you remember Doña María Apaza from chapter one, and how I told you that I'd placed her blessing into a rhodochrosite crystal heart? I want to tell you more about that rhodochrosite heart, and how to form relationships with the crystals in the mineral kingdom for your healing and well-being. In layman's terms, an in-depth explanation on how to talk to rocks! I acquired the rhodochrosite crystal only hours before I met Doña María, and its appearance was not haphazard—on the contrary, it was written in the stars. Crystals are earth's natural record keepers and the rhodochrosite crystal appeared at the perfect time to play a powerful role as a keeper of truth. In a moment of transference, I held it gently together with the flower petals of Doña María's blessing, and to this day, it holds its resonance in solid form.

When we live from the heart, we can connect with the other kingdoms that exist here on earth in a deeper way, and that means the animal kingdom, the plant kingdom, the mineral kingdom, and the elemental kingdom. Along with being the seat of compassion, the heart is also the access point to our greater self, and scientific studies are starting to reflect that. We've known since the 1800s that the heart sends more information through the nervous system to the brain than the other way around and that these signals have a huge effect on our mental clarity.[1] We also know that the heart's electromagnetic field is about sixty times greater in amplitude than that of the brain, and a hundred times stronger.[2] The heart's magnetic resonance can pick up more information than we can perceive with just the mind alone, and if we live from the heart space for long enough, the mind will recalibrate to receive its larger expression of energetic awareness.

It's been my experience that the crystal kingdom enjoys interacting with humans, and that we just need to learn how to relate to these beings in order to know this. Crystals don't speak English, but they are alive, and they do emit a frequency that reflects that aliveness. When you learned to expand into the energy of your divine inner child, you were reminded that the baseline of a heart emanating the energy of your soul is one of purity and joy. This is also true when you form a relationship with the crystal kingdom. Crystals are always emanating a high vibe output, and they don't have personal will, so it's through your ability to open your heart to joy, that brings your awareness into a space light enough to meet these beings where they are and co-create in a more conscious way. The concept in itself is easy, and I've noticed only one big fear that holds people back from testing it out—the fear of

---

1   "Scientific Foundations of the HeartMath System," HeartMath (website), YouTube Video. June 18, 2018, 2:52. https://www.heartmath.org/resources/videos/scientific-foundation-of-the-heartmath-system/

2   Rollin McCraty, *Science of the Heart Volume 2: Exploring the Role of the Heart in Human Performance*, "Chapter 6: Energetic Communication," Research Gate (PDF file), February 2016, https://www.researchgate.net/publication/293944391_Science_of_the_Heart_Volume_2_Exploring_the_Role_of_the_Heart_in_Human_Performance_An_Overview_of_Research_Conducted_by_the_HeartMath_Institute

becoming the storyline from the Christmas movie *Elf.* We are so afraid of what it would be like for our inner child to have the reins to our mind and our outward expression (especially in public), that we hold back the possibility. But with a little nudge from your inner warrior to help you through the initial unease, I'm sure you can find a way, and if you do, you'll discover a valuable skill and another part of your expression— that of a natural-born healer.

The definition of the word medicine is *a compound or preparation used for the treatment or prevention of disease*,[3] and so working with crystals as your medicine may be different in the way you experience medicine. In this case, the earth has prepared the compound, and when you allow your energy bodies to become receptive to the crystal's vibration, you are choosing to experience their treatment. The mainstream world is a society of quick fixes, fast movements, and synthetic solutions, but it has been my experience that true healing is slow moving and organic. Are you catching my drift? That crystals are highly structural codes of light and expert re-programmers of the human body? Why are the vibrations of crystals so healing? Well, from a cosmic point of view, crystals are a manifestation of light codes from the Universe that have become physically condensed into matter.[4] Just like the sun emits light rays onto the earth, there are also life-affirming vibrational rays of energy that emit onto our planet from the Universe at large. Crystals are a co-creation between the highest vibrations of cosmic light and universal love, expressing themselves in mineral form. In correlation to their high

3   "Medicine," Merriam-Webster (website), accessed February 08, 2021, https://www.merriam-webster.com/dictionary/medicine

4   Roger Calverley, *Crystal Yoga 1: The Crystal Mesa*, (Twin Lakes: Lotus Press, 2006), 171.

vibration, the psychological, emotional, and subtle physical component, each crystal will have inherent qualities of alignment, balance, and naturalness that can support us in aligning our lives back toward our naturalness.

There are many ways that you can work with crystals to support your health. Practically speaking, you can take a crystal and lay it on your forehead, chest, on your backside close to your spine, or wherever else you feel called. Healers may have a crystal wand, which they use on their clients' fields to direct and manipulate energy with precision, or grounding stones that they use themselves to stay rooted. There are such things as crystal yoni eggs that are used for womb healing, or crystal grids to create a sacred or protected space,[5] and I, personally, love to wear crystals as jewelry. The key factor to the many ways that we can relate to crystals lies in our ability to relax ourselves on a cellular level. That's because crystals are solid and structural, while humans are water-based and fluid (meaning that humans are highly programmable). When you are relaxed, your DNA expands and when your DNA is expanded, you can assimilate the resonance of the crystals' light codes into your cells to support the recoding of your DNA. All you have to do is relax and practice stilling the mind, while staying receptive, trusting, and grateful. It's like any relationship; when you come from a place of gratitude, trust, and love, you'll have a better and most likely more profound experience.

Once your inner compass has assisted you in excavating and deconstructing an old program, the time will come to replace your old program with something new. Crystals are great recruits to support you in your endeavor to

5   Nicola McIntosh, *Crystal Grid Secrets: Learn the Ancient Mysticism of Ancient Geometry*. Sydney: Rockpool Publishing, 2019.

create the energetic foundations of healthier programs. Yes, learning to relax deeply requires practice (or occasionally the support of plant medicine to temporarily relax the egoic structure), but once you become familiar with the process, these mineral beings have the power to shift your vibrational programming from their roots. In the experience of these deep vibrational shifts, you may then notice new choices, new knowledge, new opportunities, or new ways of responding to old patterns that appear out of the blue in your external world.

***

Four months before I met Doña María, I was on a coffee date with a friend. We were sitting at the open window ledge of a downtown Vancouver café, when my friend noticed that we were drinking our coffees beside a store that was owned by one of her clients. We decided to stroll over and go inside. Much to my delight, and among the other things that it sold, the store was full of crystal jewelry. It was a day of connecting, visioning, and socializing; immersed in the world of crystals, an Americano Misto at home in my belly, things were stacking up to be a five-star kind of day.

Once inside, I was like a kid in a candy shop, touching and talking about all the beautiful things. We moseyed and browsed and there at the back of the store was a rhodochrosite crystal amulet, a warm pink stone, oval, encased in silver, and decorated at the top with a small cross created from circles of raised metal. This amulet was on sale to boot. When I picked it up in my hands, the power of the crystal's offering felt like a well-known weight being dropped into the well of my heart. This stone was meant to be my medicine. So, I bought the necklace and, as was typical to my preferred way of learning, I wore it and listened. Then after a couple of weeks, I looked up the crystal's qualities to see if the findings matched up with my own.

Based on information from a book called *Crystal Yoga 1: The Crystal Mesa* by Roger Calverly (one of my favorites for sharing insight into the relationship between crystals and the growth of the soul), I discovered that rhodochrosite holds the archetypal energy of the divine child, and that it's known as the healer of hearts. Coincidence? I think not. With Soldier Al now removed from the doorway to my heart, the vibration of the rhodochrosite paired with meditation was opening up the castle doors, and I was beginning to do some housekeeping. As the days passed, the process brought into my awareness that some parts of my heart were strong, soul-centered, and full of joy, while others were huddled in the closet, scared, *terrified* for their life. And rightly so—what else is our purity to do when we come into the world like little fleshy maggots, defenseless (physically but not spiritually) to the battleground we find ourselves in? I'm grateful that Al came in to protect me from feeling the pain as a child when he did, and since I was now becoming a self-reflecting adult, wisely guiding the healing process along from a place of service to my divine inner child, I believe that same inner child had called in her second ally: the rhodochrosite amulet.

As an energy healer working with energy in a multi-dimensional way, it's often the case that my mind will spontaneously receive a download of the best solution to the issue at hand. However, a familiar frustration will often set in. My mind is very open, but since my solar plexus still needs some developing, the energetic solution will get *stuck* on its way down my central channel. From the perspective of the chakra system, it's energy that I am supposed to embody that gets stuck on its way down to earth. I am conscious of this blockage, and so when this happens

I'll sometimes bring in a crystal for support. I'll choose a stone that has the same energy signature as the energy of the solution that I need, and then place that stone onto an area of my body that is lower than my head. I assist the movement of energy by activating the same energy signature in another area; creating movement through an adjacent and attuned supportive force.

After I started to wear the rhodochrosite crystal amulet, that's exactly what happened. Many of the psychological untruths, things that I knew in my mind to be ridiculous, that still created many of the restrictions in my life (by causing me to play small), had begun to decompose before my very eyes. The freeze response that Soldier Al had been locked into all of those years, and all the pieces of experience he was protecting me from, were now melting away. As this happened, I was offered presence through the moments of pain that were undoing themselves. Conversations with my family members transformed, as I could now allow the curiosity and innocence of my divine inner child to influence new responses. Ones that were different from the patterns of my old ways, and ones that could only come about if that same inner child also had warrior protection. I noticed what would usually go unnoticed and end in tension, were now being met with a breath and a question, another breath and softness. All because it was time for some energy to move. These new ways of responding were coming from a deeper place than my intellectual will, and most excitingly they were arising without force.

After many months of wearing the rhodochrosite stone, I was grateful. In my intimate relationship with *her* (as I perceive her to be), she has worked on the inner nooks and crannies of my delicate human heart, and I was awed by her essence. She is quintessential purity, goodness, and play, and to anyone who sees otherwise, she will soften them over time with her essence of compassion. To some, purity and innocence are just a part of being naive, and that naivety is weak and something to be taken advantage of. However, naivety is only a cloak of appearance because when purity reigns in the inner realms it is the ultimate magician. It is the essence of us that can alchemize any pain and any sorrow into newness again, and as it does not dwell in pain innately, its alchemical nature propels us toward joy in every single moment. Rhodochrosite, as a master of presence and a vessel for the divine inner child, will soften our fight, melt our frozen, still our fawn, and give our flight some solid ground to stand on. The time I spent wearing my rhodochrosite amulet supported my divine inner child in a series of reclamations. And despite the emotional and at times tumultuous processing component that required me to feel *everything*, I was otherwise overjoyed. My inner world was transforming before my very eyes.

***

Let's rewind to the night I met Doña María. We are back in Mount Shasta, it's two hours before her event, and my friend Megs has taken me to visit a friend of hers. Why? Because her friend's kitchen had been transformed into a cave of crystals in every shape and size; they covered the countertop and the floors, and filled the cabinets and sinks. Each piece had been placed in position with intention and care, and I was in la-la land and ever so grateful to Megs for bringing me there. A crystal cave with pieces handpicked from around the globe and all of them were for sale, which really meant that all of them were for sharing. The crystal beings in this kitchen cave were destined for a life living in kinship with the human world.

As I moved about the room, my eyes and heart stopped at many. Some looked like they'd come straight from a dig, still clinging to the earth of the land they had grown in, while others looked as though they'd held altar space devoted to the many qualities of the divine for decades. While some of these crystals were never meant to leave those sacred walls, others waited, anxious to meet their human companion. Then I found the one meant for me, a palm sized rhodochrosite crystal heart. As crystals have their own communication system, I believe that my first crystal amulet had led me to additional support. I was in love. It was soft, flesh-like, and unassuming in nature, yet deep and electric at the same time. As I picked it up ever so sacredly, it told me that it was a Christmas gift for my mother that year.

"Wow!" says the homeowner. "You picked a wonderful one, this guy used to be a part of my personal collection. This one is from Peru."

My friend Megs pipes in, "She means it's a high-quality specimen."

"Oh, thanks," I say and explain that it will be for my mom.

The cave owner sighs, "Well isn't that nice," and holds the crystal heart in her hand for a moment of repose. "Do you have any plans for tonight?" she asks us both, realizing that I am a visitor.

Megs and I look at each other, "Nothing concrete," we respond.

"Well," replies the cave keeper, "there is a talk tonight . . . " she fumbles around as she looks for the flyer, "by a lady named Doña María at the hall, maybe you should go to that." What were the chances? I had wanted to see this woman when she'd come to visit Vancouver some months prior, but couldn't. I knew nothing about her, only that my heart had felt the call. And so, after our chill-out session in the crystal cave of wonders, we headed over to the hall, shopping bags in hand, and you know the rest.

The Rhodochrosite crystal also goes by the name of the Incan Rose, and in Incan Culture they have a myth. It's said that deep underneath the Peruvian Mountains, buried somewhere beyond our sight, there exists a massive rosy flesh colored Rhodochrosite crystal heart that holds the bloodline of the ancients, and that beats only once every 200 years. A gigantic pink crystal heart that emanates the archetypal purity and joy of the divine inner child. One massive crystal heart that beats the original heartbeat of humanity.

Chapter Fifteen:
The Magic Flower
Potion

We live in a world that is fractaline in nature. The nature of fractals is that they are infinitely the same. If you zoom in, the same design will continue to emerge, and the same goes if you were to zoom out. It's a concept that explains how the patterns we see within ourselves and within society (emotional, mental, subtle, structural, conceptual, visual, mechanical, and so on), are ones that will also be similar as we continue to expand in consciousness both internally and externally, and into what is beyond the current perception of our ego (meaning into other densities of life).

Each human vessel is also like a radio transmitter. As much as we are a node of fractality, we are also giving and receiving information, and how we interpret that information is based on our foundational programs. You have learned that when you change your programming, it means that your life will change as well. At the deepest level this change happens through energetics, yet it can also be witnessed from our outer layers too. For example, a mutation to a cell in the body, a change to a word in a sentence spoken, or any action taken in a change of course, is a fractal expression that is changing forwards and backwards into time. In an arraying manner rather than in a linear one, that change will then affect the experience of those beings who are around it.

Consciousness is also infinite and expanding, and much of what exists is beyond the capacity of our human intelligence to comprehend. Yet, we are evolving, and as our egos expand past third density awareness, we'll naturally interpret what's new to us in a way that is similar to our node of fractaline perception. You are now learning that on the other side of the veil, there is not a black void of nothingness. Instead, there is just more information, and since humans are the most fulfilled when they are on purpose and learning through love, it's to our benefit if we choose to interpret that new information from the heart, and through a lens that is safe, enjoyable, and digestible to us.

Being a fractaline radio transmitter living from the heart brings us to another new concept: that of **spirit guides**. We all have guides beyond the veil whose job is to care specifically for us. Maybe you're already familiar with the idea of angels watching over us, or messages from God, and through a new paradigm lens we are now going to make a few tweaks to this concept. The most significant change, when we wake up to our connection to the other side, is that what's beyond the veil becomes more sophisticated.[1] We discover that there are layers of hierarchy and a multiplicity of beings who exist in the non-physical world (angels, extraterrestrials, souls who are not incarnated at this time, deceased loved ones, ascended masters, archangels, and also demons—so we must be discerning) and if they are connected to earth it means they have a job to do (with

1 Barbara Y. Martin, *Communing with the Divine: A Clairvoyant's Guide to Angels, Archangels, and the Spiritual Hierarchy.* New York: Jeremy P. Tarcher, 2014.

us). The second tweak is that those jobs become more personalized, as each of us is assigned a guide or two, who's main purpose is to guide us through life. Their main assignment is making sure we stay on track with what we incarnated to learn, and if we practice connecting to them through our hearts, these relationships can become a co-creation (making them all that much more fun for everyone). As you are learning how to awaken your HSP, you might also consider making a connection to your guides.

Connecting to your spirit guides is your next assignment, while in this case, it's not a mandatory one. If expanding your ego in this way makes you feel scared, consider holding off for now, while if the thought makes you feel excited, why not dive right in! The first step is to set your intention to connect and say, "I would like to connect to my benevolent and divinely contracted spirit guides," which should do the trick (three times in a row is even more powerful). Next, try writing in a journal about what you'd like guidance on, and let your mind become open to receiving the answers as you walk through your daily life. The easiest way to start is to look for and notice repeating numbers (which you can look up online to find the meaning of), signs, and inner nudges, and as you become more advanced it can become as literal as hearing their voice in your head, or through images they project into your mind's eye. Now would be a good time to take a nice big breath, and see how you feel in your heart about what you are reading. Take in what works for you and leave the rest behind, drink some water and let any new information settle. If you resonate with what you've just read, maybe you want to get up and dance it through to let it in. Or simply take a moment to notice and honor how you are feeling, how your heart is beating, and breathe.

***

One day, I noticed that I had a new fascination with an old memory. It was one of an energy healing session where I was the client, and where Megs was the practitioner. At this time, I was devoutly invested (as I still am now) in knowing why my heart, or the muscles and nerves around the area of my heart, felt numb. During the session, in my mind's eye, I saw a vivid image of a room full of beautiful furniture in mint condition, and I understood that these pieces of furniture had maintained their integrity because they were protected by a plastic covering. The plastic, however, was covered in dust and debris to a level that said they'd been there for centuries. Centuries of untouched, unseen, majestic furniture, representing my protected, yet unseen, untouched, and majestic heart. At that time, the lesson I received was patience. The budding heart warrior within me learned that it was the covering around her heart that held the pain, and that for now patience was her medicine. I was asked to slow down.

After I remembered this vision and its meaning, I then felt the need to walk over to my bookshelf and take out an old book. It was called *Natural Healing Wisdom and Know-How* by Amy Rost, a book that I hadn't looked at in years. As is usual for my spirit guides to do, they then flipped me directly to the page I needed. A page on Bach Flower Remedies and into a world of healing created by Dr. Edward Bach. Dr. Bach knew that the vibrations of flowers naturally corresponded to different parts of the human body, and that we could administer them using acupressure points.

Acupressure points are pressure points on the body's surface that connect into the meridian lines that run throughout the body's interior. Making up the major pathways in the etheric body, meridian lines are energy highways of light that distribute information, our body's exclusive postal network. Dr. Bach understood that by placing the vibrational essence of a flower onto its corresponding acupressure point, we could transfer the flower's vibration to a specific location. Flower essences are another realm of earth's subtle magic and like the crystals, we work with them in a non-invasive, very kind, and gentle way.

The page I was opened to spoke about the pericardium: known as the heart protector, it's a sac of protective membrane that surrounds the heart. In other words, the dusty plastic covering's anatomical twin. My third ally had come forward. It was the Agrimony flower, and its resonant acupressure point was located in the middle of my forearm, just above my wrist. Now that I had created a structural shift with the crystals, the Agrimony flower was going to help it bloom by opening the castle doors, turning on the lights to what was inside, and removing the debris-filled plastic from my ancient heart.

According to the book that I was guided to open, "The pericardium acts as the doorway into your heart, and it allows you to access your most intimate feelings. This is the site to use when the gate to your heart has been shut. Bringing a feeling of protective warmth, it gives you the courage to see the damage that has occurred and helps you begin speaking your truth again. Applying Agrimony **flower essence** to the inner frontier gate enables light from the world to flood the inner sanctum of your heart, restoring joy."[2]

I sat for a moment, astonished by the precision of the book's message. It was true, my heart had been locked down from the world. Yes, I had spent the last seven years

2   Amy Rost and Rachel Hasna, *Natural Healing Wisdom & Know How: Useful Practices, Recipes, and Formulas for a Lifetime of Health,* (New York: Black Dog & Leventhal Publishers, 2017), 289.

getting to know myself, and I did love myself quite a bit. But, even though I knew myself intimately, no one else really did. They knew parts of me, but as I had learned to live in humanity's chronic separation from its souls' light, what should have naturally been a momentary shield (freeze response) between the world and my authenticity, had instead become a permanent fixture. My truest self became concealed behind thick castle doors, and with the defense of a guard my spiritual self remained hidden quietly waiting to be seen. But now I was evolving, and through a series of small, yet courageous choices, I was giving myself permission to shine.

AGRIMONY ESSENCE PRESCRIPTION

Apply a light pulsing pressure to the inner frontier gate acupressure point, intending for the gate to open. With your forearm held in a horizontal position, place five drops of Agrimony Essence twice daily and rest in this position for five to ten minutes. While practicing presence throughout the process, use your intention to guide the directive and infuse love.

Crystals and flowers to heal Alzheimer's disease? That is probably not what you expected this book to conclude with, yet my answer to this serious question is both no . . . and yes. In Western medicine, the definition of the word disease is "a state in which there has been sufficient departure from the normal for signs and symptoms to be produced,"[3] while the term Alzheimer's

---

3   David Li Lam, *The Basic Anatomy & Physiology for Bodywork Practitioners: Study Notes,* (Vancouver: Langara College Continuing Studies, 2018), 15.

is named after its discoverer—Dr. Alois Alzheimer. So technically, Alzheimer's disease means that there has been enough toxic build-up in the brain to cause nerve death and noticeable memory loss. In this case, since I didn't yet show any symptoms, the answer to the question I posed is no, crystals and flowers don't heal Alzheimer's. Instead, what I am suggesting in this book, as investigated so far, is that it can reverse it during an earlier timeline where the physical symptoms are yet to be expressed. This more mystical (yet still, scientific) approach is currently doing vibrational work on the layers of my consciousness to subtly change the fractaline nature of my expression, which came online to be discovered when my soul-self called me home.

So, this is where the yes comes in. Yes, I wholeheartedly embraced a relationship with the crystals and the flowers as healers on my path, and if that makes me a quintessential flower child in your eyes, I will gladly accept. That's because my flower child actions connect me to something, which, I feel, is profound and universal, and it's this: we are not separate from nature, and when we come home to her, we heal.

If the earth was left up to her own prerogative, we would see that health and wellness are in the essence of the oceans and trees, the rainforests and mushrooms, and the flowers and ecosystems that form the continents. When we learn to pay attention, and when we feel the call to heal in a way that comes through from a soul-centered heart, we discover that mother earth has all the remedies and she provides them to us because we are her children. She is the archetypal essence of humanity's beautiful mother. She loves us unconditionally, immeasurably, and innately, and she is always there, patiently waiting for us to listen.

Chapter Sixteen:
An Exclusive
on Fear

The earth vibrates with love, goodness, abundance, and power . . . so where exactly does fear fit into the equation? What is the purpose of fear? And are there different kinds? This chapter is dedicated to the first question while to the second and third I say, *yes* there are different kinds of fear, and there are some things that fear is good for, and some things that it is not. There is natural fear: the kind that animals feel when they are being hunted, or the jolt we get as a car zooms by right before we cross the street. It is the momentary fear that comes from our nervous system when we feel that our life is being threatened. In chapter ten, you also learned that fear can be covert, and that we can get stuck in fear-based patterns that become possible when we move away from presence.

We also feel fear when our egos are reaching the end of their domain. It is natural for our ego to fight to the death inducing fear, until we break through to the other side of its borders. This is the fear we get when we are about to do a big presentation, make a new choice, break down an old belief, or ask a big question. It's a healthy way for our being to tell us *hey we are doing something entirely new here.* If we acknowledge that fear and then walk through it (in a healthy amount of time), we are saying yes to expansion and growth, which is an ideal response.

The last type of fear that I've noticed and the one that I am going to talk about here is untethered fear. This is the fear we see broadcasted on the news, or through a story passed on from our neighbor. It's the type of fear that is no longer located in the same moment as the events that created it, and because it's untethered, it is highly contagious, and spreads like wildfire through word of mouth.

As an energy sensitive person, when fear arises I feel it like an icy white-silver electric charge that sparks up my aura, enters my chakras, and causes me to contract. I have two great stories that I want to share about untethered fear, and before I tell them, I first want to acknowledge that fear, when you're feeling it at the moment, is a powerful and all encompassing emotion. I know that when fear has gotten a hold, it's a hard emotion to shake.

The first story comes to you from my time spent in India. I rented a moped while I was there, and I adventurously drove on the streets. Do you know what else drives on the streets of India? Cows, cars, motorcycles, trucks, wagons, elephants, and rickshaws, and unless you have a local's vision, there are layers of madness before you get any sense of method into what's going on as far as road rules go. It was a total event to get myself to school or to go out for a spin, and always visually stimulating. Eventually, I started to play a game; the instructions I learned from the most rebellious *or* the most quick-minded of the locals. At stoplights, with all the above-mentioned characters involved, I learned to weave my way through the crowd with the aim of getting to the front before the light turned green. It was *Frogger,* traffic jam edition, and extremely thrilling (while going three kilometers an hour).

I learned the streets, and over time I would even say I became comfortable with them. I also noticed that when I told my native friends that I drove, I always seemed to receive the same response. Not only that, but I was told over and over, and with much conviction, that I should *never* drive at night. At first, I would kindly acknowledge their caution, but as I noticed the narrative recurring, I also started to ask, "Why?" The funny thing was that no one seemed to have an answer, other than, "That someone had told them so."

One night, after some friends and I had gone out dancing, I had a firm sense that arose within saying it was time to go home. It also happened to be very late. Yet, when I listened to my instincts, which existed underneath the fear, they told me it was an impulse and that it was safe to go home. So, with a higher dose of boldness and a few less wrinkles than I have now, I declared to my friends that, contrary to popular belief, I felt sure of my safety and that I would drive myself home. I left the party in the early morning hours, and do you know what I discovered on the other side of my classmates' fear? Silence. Sleeping dogs who freckled the streets and stillness. I learned that there was a sense of peace and solitude that existed in the middle of the night in India. Amidst the daily bustle of a dense population filled with the sounds of horns honking and people jabbering, it was a silence that could not be found in any other moment. If I had not listened to my inner knowing, I would never have known it to exist. As a young twenty-something-year-old who still gave her power away to authority, I got home safe and sound that night, and acquired a revelation through this experience. I learned that I could trust myself, and I activated more of my personal power because of it. That night taught me to listen to my inner knowing, and that I could refuse a message from untethered fear if that's what I wanted to do.

My second story happened just a few years back when I traveled to the Pyrenees mountains in France. In a month of adventuring, I had scheduled three stops. The first was a spiritual tour of the sacred places of Mary Magdalene. Here our base camp was a little bed-and-breakfast full of French bread and cheese, that doubled as a sacred feminine temple. The second was a work stay at a mushroom farm, located along the winding road of a remote mountainside hamlet. Here I stayed in an old cabin with little hot water and breathtaking views. The third was just a mountain side where I trained to spend three days alone in the wilderness. A tarp, a sleeping bag, and a master cleanse diet were my only supplies. I spent the first week touring the sacred places of Mary Magdalene, checking out ancient churches, and sacred caves and sites. In our little group of five, we spent time philosophizing and searching for the holy grail. In the second week at the mushroom farm, I learned how to grow mushrooms in both outdoor and indoor environments, and helped to rebuild the foundations of a very old mountainside barn. During the last week on the wilderness solo, after two days of preparation, I spent time contemplating my existence on the side of a rolling mountain's ridge.

During the second phase of my adventure, I had the complete pleasure of watching a vast flock of sheep trail up the mountainside with their shepherds. It sure was something, all the bells and the baaing, and sheepdogs doing their work. As they stopped at our through passage, the older sheep lay down to rest, like they knew the drill from years of practice. While the shepherds stopped to say *bonjour*, they told us an unfortunate tale of a local who had been trampled and killed by a mother cow. A tragic story of a man who had fatefully positioned himself between a mother and her baby (in distress). There it was again, untethered fear, and this time I felt it enter my system like wisps of silver-grey electricity coming into my field from all angles, and then a contraction. This conversation took place on the side of a mountain where seven people lived. With no televisions and no wifi, the lack of synthetic stimulation created more room for insight into my organic experience.

The shaman in me chose to spend the last week of my vacation on a vision quest—I was soon to be thirty, and I decided it was time for a heart-to-heart. During my time isolated from everything but nature's embrace, can you guess who I had as my honored guests? That's right, cows. Many, many cows. The mountains of my wilderness solo were part of a farm, and evidently, I had chosen to camp right beside the passage of its cows' daily commute. In the summer months as a child, I grew up feeding baby cows on my grandparents' dairy farm. I never developed a close kinship to them, but I also never experienced fear when I went for visits. Cows are commonly known as docile creatures, so imagine my surprise when I reacted to their presence on the mountainside in the following manner.

In my response to these docile creatures approaching, I discovered myself scrambling up the side of the mountain in the scorching sun so that I could hide at the top of a little rock cliff. My heart was racing, and I thought to myself, *oh my gosh, why am I so afraid of cows?* Images of my death raced through my mind, and I considered what I would do if one of them charged.

Lost in thought, I watched in a haze as they licked my small backpack, their cowbells clanging deep brassy tones, tails flicking in the breeze. Some of them looked up at me, considering my presence on their journey, and as they did, I acknowledged that they were inquisitive, and not angry. My thoughts then shifted to hoping that none of them would do their business near my sleeping quarters.

As I sat there hunched on my sunny rock cliff, cycling through sitting positions, so that no one part of my body would feel like it was being burnt, I laughed at the absurdity of my situation, and acknowledged the strength of fear's capacities to make things in our lives more difficult for us.

Like I said at the beginning of this chapter, fear can happen as a natural response to when our body feels unsafe, like when we stand near the edge of a cliff or contemplate walking down a dark alley, or even if someone is thinking bad thoughts about us. Fear gives us a read on the situation at hand, and so it is good practice to notice if the objects, scenarios, or beings in the fearful narrative you are running, are with you in the present moment. If they are not, most likely you have a case of untethered fear on your hands. This type of fear can steal your power and greatly disrupt the healing process on all levels. So, do your best to notice, take a breath, reset, and say thank you. Then imagine it for what it really is, just wisps of silver energy that need your life force in order to stay alive.

Chapter Seventeen: Alzheimer's and the Soul

Each human is their very own personal universe, and perhaps after reading all that you've just read, you can now see the true beauty of what that universe really is! This is your beauty, an all-encompassing expression of every breath you've ever taken, every feeling you've ever felt, every thought you've ever thought, and every action you've ever acted—all held in your aura and then condensed into physical form. As a soul who is the master of its universe, you have the birthright to claim loving responsibility for everything you experience, perhaps more deeply than what you previously thought possible. All the characters you've ever played over lifetimes are equal to the expansion you now embody on a soul level. As you practice treating the imbalances you find (which have been created innocently through unconsciousness) as noble lessons—like battle wounds from your soul's life in the matrix—it's then that you can sink deep enough to create soul-based transformation.

The current paradigm we live in is dualistic and polarized, like a checkerboard or a scale of justice. While humans have a soul nature, which innately unifies them with what's around them, the architects at the highest levels of this paradigm are committed to propagating a divide, as this is the type of matrix they feel comfortable living in.

I hope that the thickest thread in this book is one which teaches that human beings are innately based in love. Perhaps this was something that you already knew, only needing a gentle reminder. On the other hand, this next statement may be something that you don't yet know, and the reason I placed the seeds of alien experiences in the previous chapters. I wanted to introduce you to the galactic perspective.

While the human race is innately based in love, most of the people at the very top of our world systems are not indigenous human souls (although they may look human), and the current paradigm is theirs. Their naturalness is not the same as our naturalness, and they maintain their livelihood through the friction, struggle, and suffrage in human conflict. They are covertly devoted to creating the very same world chaos that they are also outwardly devoted to helping the world solve. War, greed, rape, the aggressor, and the victim, are all natural to their innate essence, while the purity of a creative and joyful child, is the foundation of ours.

Have you ever considered the reason why we live in such a pyramidal structure? Who really is at the top of it all? The truth is daunting, but the good news is that there are many of us and few of them. Learning the fullness of this structure is another stage of awakening, as darkness cannot exist in the light of awareness.

I called the world we live in a false light matrix because when we break through its glass ceiling we have a new ability to see the fullness of its structure. This is a vision, which sees the conflict and the resolution as two sides of the same coin. Through masterful trickery we have been hooked, and in our innocence (and over centuries) we have consented. Paradoxically, it's the very same innocence innate to our species that will undo us from it. It's when we choose to move back toward our innocence that we gain the epoch of wisdom of our soul's many lives living in the matrix. It's a powerful move to make the distinction between human and non-human souls in our vision because we'll no longer be fooled into pointing the finger at each other when our mainstream culture so craftily invites us to do so. We will have learned to see their trickery for what it is, and as we each awaken in our own divine timing, we'll have the ability to release ourselves from their trauma-based programs (if that's what we choose to do).

There is also another vantage point to embrace because the closer we get to the atman of our nature, the more we can claim the other as something within us. From this vantage point, we see those alien impulses as something innately in us as well. This is the level of awareness that claims each battle as an inner battle, and each joy an inner joy. As the old epoch closes, just like a diamond whose beauty has been created through pressure, our souls have been through the pressure of this matrix, and it's the reason we have grown into the resilient species that we are today. As we move forward into the new era, each lesson we complete assists us in excavating our diamond nature in order to live unbounded.

***

I have come across some interesting stories in my time spent studying Alzheimer's and the soul, and the first one comes from a healer named Mark Bajerski, who shares his experience assisting a man with Alzheimer's on his YouTube channel.[1] In his story, he describes how his client was brought to his sessions by his wife. Mark would place his hands on his client, allow divine energy

1   Mark Bajerski, "Alzheimer's and Dementia, What's Really Happening Spiritually. The Bigger Picture," YouTube Video, 1:15. June 26, 2018, https://www.youtube.com/watch?v=bIqjHZ2sdaY

to channel through him, and then he would sense his client's soul coming back into its body. The client and his wife would then leave the session in the same state as they came, but after a couple of days the client's wife would report to Mark that her husband had returned. At first, the man's soul would stay for weeks, but always it would leave again and each time this happened, the man's wife would take him back in to see Mark. As they repeated this process, the man's soul would proceed to stay for shorter and shorter amounts of time, until finally, it wouldn't come back at all.

Similarly, I know of a healer who can remove cancerous tumors from the human body, but she also explained to me this: it's often the case that if the client doesn't invest in learning the lessons and healing in a holistic way, that the cancer will grow back, and on its third occurrence it becomes nearly impossible for the cancer to be removed. The energy the client's biofield had invested in removing the cancer would have depleted the client's power, which allowed the cancer's growth and lethality to increase when it returned.

These are just two examples of more radical healing experiences that resonated with me as I spent time studying and learning, and the message they share is the same as mine. If we don't learn the lessons, we won't heal in a deep enough way to create lasting changes. That's why I've chosen a template that takes you to the root. I've also chosen to share with you what I've discovered while investigating my own roots as well. However, the underlying reason why an illness will manifest has details that are unique to each of us. What's the same is the zero point potential in our hearts from where all possibilities stem. Each one of us is powerful beyond measure, and I wish for you to feel this truth as much as I do in your own way. Otherwise, not even a healer can help you shift and transform the programs that exist in the deeper parts of you, to remove them from their roots. Only we can do that for ourselves—but loving support is always available in the process.

The final link in our journey together is to make the connection between our physical biology and the codes in our energy fields. Before I considered writing this book, the medical world remained a foreign terrain. In my early years, I gave my power away to doctors unquestionably; after my awakening, I moved away from that world, trading in pills for breath-work, combatting symptoms with shifts in my diet, and facing the fear of pain with a holistic embrace. Until now, Western medicine had yet to integrate into my personal world, but in order to write this book the way I envisioned it, I needed to give Western medicine a second look.

What I found was an interesting surprise, as I felt the world of medical academia to be one of optimistic discovery and fiery passion, where advanced technological tools allow us to look at the human body in a profound degree of detail. It's a field that has created an astonishing moving map of the body's physicality and biology, and allowed me to explore the translation of human consciousness into its microscopic physical form.

The Toxic Build Up of Plaques and Tangles: In the physical domain, the hallmark build up of plaques and tangles in Alzheimer's disease is created by two types of naturally occurring proteins that accumulate in the brain to an unnatural level. Compellingly, the word proteins is derived from the Greek word *proteios* meaning "the first quality."[2] So, what dynamic in the life of an

2   "Protein," Online Etymology Dictionary (website), accessed February 08, 2021, https://www.etymonline.com/word/protein

incarnated soul would have caused them to accumulate too much of some "first quality" in their mind, causing that first quality to become toxic?

Since we know the world to be polarized, and in connection with this truth, we can assume that when we step away from our health, we step away from balance. Illness suggests that a soul is likely living a life, has lived a life, or a series of lives in more extreme versions of polarization (usually in an unconscious way) and has yet to reconcile those polarities through the heart. There are also exceptions to this rule, as sometimes a soul will choose a lifetime with illness because the lessons they'll be learning are more valuable to them than their health. Often, it's through adversities that we evolve the most.

In Alzheimer's, proteins accumulate in the brain (consider that subtle energy is being inputted through your third eye chakra to become microscopic pieces of matter over time), until they reach a tipping point. The physical ecosystem of a brain with Alzheimer's is one where small proteins called β-amyloid peptide accumulate in the synapses (the gap between where neurons meet to transfer the electrical impulses of data that create thoughts and memories), to such a level that our microglia cells (those cells whose role it is to clean up these plaques) are unable to keep up with the peptide accumulation, and the clearing process becomes hyper-activated and inflamed. This inflammation is then linked to the activation of the enzyme kinase which causes the tau protein, a naturally occurring protein in the cytoskeleton of the neuron (the structural wall of the cell), to change in shape, which creates neurofibrillary tangles (tau protein clumped together). This clumping affects the integrity of the cell wall, which is what causes neuron death (inhibiting the transfer of electrical impulses that create and store memories) in progresive regions of the brain over time.[3]

From a soul level, what conditions would be needed to create this toxic build up around the third eye? While it's true that the personal expression of the dis-ease will be unique to each of us, we can also explore Alzheimer's in its archetypal form: a way of living where the use of the mind greatly outweighs the intelligence of the heart. Deeper still is the condition that this book was dedicated to, for someone to become disconnected from the inner compass of their soul. In a world that lives in its outer being, this is a condition that happens to so many of us, and creates the predisposition for a soul to stay in environments that are unhealthy to it. Our minds are masters at rationalizing reasons we should stay in situations, even if they don't feel good.

As this imbalance is created, a polarity develops in our psyches, and that tends to create two different types of people: those who output energy through power and those who output energy through powerlessness. You may know it by its more common titles as the narcissist and the co-dependent,[4] or the victim and the aggressor. In the word of energy, you could say that a narcissist is someone who is always outputting their energy with authority, while drawing in the energy of those around them in return; and the co-dependent is someone who is always giving away their energy through servitude, while drawing in the energy of those around them in return. It's the naturalness of a subtle heart that gives and receives (inhales and exhales), while

3   "What Happens to the Brain in Alzheimer's Disease?" National Institute on Aging (website), last reviewed May 16, 2017, https://www.nia.nih.gov/health/what-happens-brain-alzheimers-disease.

4   Melody Beattie, *Codependent No More & Beyond Codependency*. New York: MJF Books, 1992.

still in service to the power structures of our third density world. A dynamic that is created when we haven't yet remembered our innate worth, or how to replenish our lives from the inside out through the elixir of our soul.

Professor Margaret Rogers Van Coops, in her podcast, "Journey into an Unknown World,"[5] explains Alzheimer's to be the expression of someone who has gotten caught up supporting others, without realizing that their deeper desire is a call from their soul for them to support themselves. The development of Alzheimer's then is thought to be the expression of an unmet need in those who are living unconscious to their inner world, and so continue to meet their program's impulse in a way that only reaches as deep as their outer being. Thus, setting the stage for those incarnated souls to accumulate toxicity from their external environment over time.

This accumulation of toxicity can be created in multiple ways, but they all stem from a lack of awareness of what it would feel like to exist on a higher vibration of holistic well-being. Do you remember in chapter seven how I said that the odds have been stacked against us for quite some time? I was referring to the mechanics of the old paradigm. The world at present is inundated with subtleties that are toxic to the typical organic human, but they can also be overridden as we learn the power of our alchemical nature. To most of us, however, these subtleties go unacknowledged and because we remain unaware they are effectively micro-dosing us over time. These toxicities can come in forms such as chemtrails, GMOs, wifi, emotional stresses, toxic thoughts, and so on. This micro-dosing is then worsened as we traverse the world disconnected from grounding to our Mother Earth (which creates a

---

5   Margaret Rogers Van Coops, "Journey into an Unknown World-Appreciate Your Brain," Podcast Addict. September 4, 2017, 28:00. https://podcastaddict.com/episode/116468111

natural detoxing circuit), and at a pace that is too quick for our body's natural healing abilities to keep up with. And all of this is innocent, as most of us are not yet taught the importance of holistic well-being.

Anger and the Death of our Nerve Cells: The neuroscientist Lisa Genova, during her TED Talk on Alzheimer's describes, "β-amyloid plaques as a lit match, at the tipping point the match sets fire to the forest."[6] As I listened to her talk, I noticed a parallel between this biological process she explains so well, and the emotional signature of the disease that energy healer Mark Bajerski refers to as its trademark. He describes the typical pattern of Alzheimer's to be one of, "Something's gotta give, something's gotta blow (perhaps inadvertently describing the emotional level of the cleaning, inflammation, cytoskeleton deterioration, and neurons' death cycle). When you are in the frustration of worry, fear, and anger, it's like you're sticking your foot down on the accelerator in a vehicle and the wheels are spinning. But the vehicle is raised, so nothing is happening. You're not going anywhere, but you're burning, burning . . . and you can smell the burning until eventually the engine blows, and it gives up."[7] I find this to be an insightful example of how the different dimensions of our expression reflect and co-exist in a holistic way. Mark's recount gives insight into the power of our emotional body and the effect that it has on our physical expression. It's an example of where our emotional expressions go (into the body), and how they affect our biology if we aren't taught how to embrace them in the

---

6   Lisa Genova, "What You Can Do to Prevent Alzheimer's," Filmed April 2017 in Vancouver, BC. TED video, 13:48. https://www.ted.com/talks/lisa_genova_what_you_can_do_to_prevent_alzheimer_s?language=en

7   Bajerski, "Alzheimer's and Dementia."

moments when they arise (which should effectively create a change of course in our lives).

The next story comes from *The Nun Study* by David A. Snowdon; an inspiring scientific study that throws a curveball in our conventional understanding of what Alzheimer's disease assumes to be. Written in 1995 and published in the *Gerontologist* in 1997,[8] the study highlights a nun named Sister Mary who demonstrated healthy cognitive test scores before her death at 101, despite ranking in the top ten percent of her study group for the classic lesions of Alzheimer's disease. Snowdon suggests that the anomaly of Sister Mary's situation could be caused by the atypical distribution of plaques and tangles in her brain (as her neocortex showed significantly less damage than the rest of her peers, while the hippocampus showed significantly more). What stood out to me, however, was the holistic nature of the study as it remarked on Sister Mary's obvious aliveness as much as it analyzed the data which was derived later through an autopsy. The author described Sister Mary as having, "eyes that radiated joy and peace . . . and a warm and hearty cackle of a laugh that boomed out of her room at all hours of the day and night."[9]

The study also included this quote from Sister Mary's memorial service, "and what was the secret to her longevity? I remember her telling me that one day she had wondered out loud to her doctor if perhaps he was giving her medicine to keep her alive, and after all, she desired to be with Jesus. Her doctor replied, 'Sister, it's not my medicine that's keeping you alive. It's your attitude!' And it was that wonderful attitude that we all loved. It was that

---

8   David A. Snowdon, "Aging and Alzheimer's Disease: Lessons From the Nun Study," *The Gerontologist* 37, no. 2 (April 1997): 150-156. https://doi.org/10.1093/geront/37.2.150

9   Snowdon, "Aging and Alzheimer's Disease," 151.

attitude that St. Paul describes so well of wanting and not wanting to remain on earth. We all know how much Sister Mary longed for heaven, but we all saw how alert and involved she was in what was going on around her. She was there in the present moment with all her heart and soul."[10] These touching remarks on Sister Mary's disposition caused me to wonder this: In the world of spirit, could it be that the aliveness from a soul whose joy and compassion has grown abundantly into the present moment, trumps the reality of the body's physical conditions? Perhaps this was also the same level of joy and compassion that touched me through the blessing I received from Doña María.

It is largely considered in esoteric wisdom that the soul incarnates into the heart (also anchoring in the solar plexus and the sacral chakra), and then permeates outwards, encompassing the entire body and aura. Perhaps it is for those among us who are much more spiritually evolved (doctorate-level souls) that the power of their soul as it embraces the physical body is much more sophisticated than we realize. In Sister Mary's case, it appears to be that her soul was especially present in life, and as a result could override the body's physical symptoms.

In its more typical expression, the subtle-spiritual component of Alzheimer's disease is one where the soul has loosened its anchoring from the body, and as it does this I noticed a strong correlation between the disease's symptoms, and the deterioration of the lower three layers of the auric field over time. You are now someone who is aware of how the layers of the aura develop in a child as they grow, so try imagining those layers deteriorating backward in those among us who are experiencing Alzheimer's disease.

---

10   Snowdon, "Aging and Alzheimer's Disease," 150.

LAYER OF THE AURIC FIELD	SYMPTOMS[11]
The Third Layer of the Field: Deterioration of the Mental Body.	Difficulty remembering new information. Difficulty understanding and communicating. Difficulty making decisions, performing simple tasks, and following conversations. Spatial impairment and losing their way. Experience of memory loss, initially for recent events and eventually for long-term events.
The Second Layer of the Field: Deterioration of the Emotional Body.	Mood and behavior changes, apathy towards things they once loved. Some become less expressive and withdrawn. Some relive old memories.
The First Layer of the Field: Deterioration of the Etheric Body.	Reduced coordination and mobility functions, to the point of affecting the ability to perform day-to-day tasks such as eating, bathing, getting dressed, and walking. Shutting down of the heart and lungs.

Our soul nature speaks most strongly to us through metaphor and poetry, and the higher parts of who we are have a way of seeing everything that exists as divine perfection birthing itself anew in every moment.

11 *Symptoms List Source:* "Alzheimer's Disease," Alzheimer's Society of Huron County, updated October 4, 2019, https://alzheimer.ca/en/huroncounty/About-dementia/Alzheimer-s-disease

I pondered this thought as I sat at a Starbucks one afternoon finishing my school essay, and I asked my guides, "Why Alzheimer's? And why is it on the rise?" After I posed these questions in my mind, I immediately began to cry, and that's how I knew they were sharing something important with me. The world really is evolving, and we are all a part of this evolutionary jump. As a soul, it could mean incarnating into another planetary system in your next incarnation, or it could mean choosing to do the work of raising your vibration in this one. One thing is for sure, to stay in alignment with the earth as she shifts into a higher density, the human species is also required to rise in awareness, while so much in our environment (alterations to our food, water, air, etc.) inhibit this rise. Because of this, not all humans are capable of becoming conscious co-creators of their personal shift in this lifetime. It will likely be that the older we are, the more densified an outer being we will have, and there are many souls who are not yet strong enough to break through the illusions of the matrix. Yet, many of these earth souls are also souls who still desire to stay in alignment with the earth's shift, and I believe that the experience of Alzheimer's disease (as there are negative and positive perspectives to every situation in polarity) can help to facilitate this.

When we choose to live from a soul-centered heart, we will be called to integrate and expand through our trauma-based relational patterns. To do this, we will likely have to become both sides in our inner world in order to be successful. I believe that Alzheimer's can be a situational expansion from this truth, as it offers a unique opportunity for relational healing to take place in our family units. As our loved ones progress, their mind loses its power. The silver lining in this truth is that so does their conditioning and the masks they have worn, which have helped to keep their unprocessed pain neatly tucked away within.

If the caretakers of those who are experiencing Alzheimer's practice resting in presence as they are care-taking, I believe that they can witness releases from the soul, as deeply buried truths become revealed. Mood and behavioral changes are a known symptom of Alzheimer's, and now that you have some new theories to understand the wholeness of your human nature, see if you can hold space for those emotions differently. As generational patterns get revealed, you might even gain insight into pieces of your family line that you have yet to know. The level of vulnerability that losing our mind offers is the type of insight that can break the chain of unconscious trauma, and create epic shifts for generations to come.

Karma: During my awakening, there was a moment when I asked, "Why am I here again?" *Here* being earth, and the answer that came through my lips in the next moment was, "Karma." Karma was the reason I returned, because to process the karma I had created on earth, I needed to be on location. This, I believe, is another positive component of Alzheimer's: The soul now has one foot in this world and one foot in the other—a creative way of bypassing the rigidity of the mind to process karma. For those souls who leave a portion of themselves (their physical vessel) on the earth plane, they hold on to this ability to process earthly karma, and in these times of epic changes, that's really a great thing. Karma held inside of families now has the opportunity to be witnessed and understood uniquely as family members learn to intimately meet the needs of their loved ones. This occurs when their loved ones lose the ability to meet their needs themselves.

For those family members who are care-taking their parents or aging relatives, consider that the soul of your loved one is still closely navigating what they can from the fourth density of the astral plane. To connect with their soul-self, allow love to expand into your dynamic; this might mean softening, letting go of expectations, resting into the present moment, or seeking a dose of higher wisdom as you practice living with a heart that's full through day-to-day tasks. In the most difficult of times, remember that you have loving guides from the higher spiritual realms at your side to support you. You and your loved ones are irreplaceable in the eyes of God and if you need support, all you have to do is ask.

A Soul Fracture that Leaves the Body Behind: A soul fracture is when a piece of our soul energy has become separated from our soul's conscious experience. In the same way that traumas of this lifetime are aspects of us that have separated from our conscious experience, soul fractures are created from the experiences we've had in other lives that we have yet to process and integrate. They are pieces of us that remain locked in time until we become conscious of how to integrate them. On a soul level, the opportunity for lineage healing is a positive side to Alzheimer's, while a negative side is a predisposition for a new soul fracture to be formed. This can happen as the layers of the field deteriorate and the biofield loses its ability to process life's new experiences. Do you remember how a small child will need an adult close by to support them to co-regulate their emotions? Well, I believe that those experiencing Alzheimer's may need the same assistance as they advance in the expression of their disease. This is something that becomes possible when we learn to care-take through presence and curiosity (instead of through fear and contraction).

An intuitive healer named Abbey Normal does a fantastic job of interpreting the experience of a soul who is in the advanced stages of Alzheimer's disease.[12] Her intuitive interpretation supports the importance of giving love to the body of those who are in the later stages of the disease's progression. Things like loving the body through touch, a gentle hand held at the back of the heart chakra, and caressing the skin of your loved one's face, can become some of the most healing actions of your care-taking role. Just like a baby who's newly born into this world, those in the advanced stages of Alzheimer's no longer have an aura to protect them, and so we should aim to support the body of our loved ones with the same loving embrace. If you are the caregiver of someone experiencing Alzheimer's, instead of thinking about the details of this or that, try thinking about the overall tone of your loved one's experience. Aim for it to be safe, simple, and full of connection from people who care. Since the soul's connection to its etheric body is the last layer of awareness to leave, consider the care-taking of the body as your biggest focus.

The moment I became aware that the soul of Ms. J was traveling, was the moment I wanted to share this information with the world. I expect there are many people who are clouded in the pain and fear of where their loved one has gone, and it doesn't have to be this way because the soul of your loved one is eternal and untouched by the temporality of this world. A soul-based approach to Alzheimer's gives us new insight into why toxic proteins build up in the mind, but then some new questions arise: Why is it that the soul can split from its body when the deterioration of the mind and mental body occur? Why

---

12   Abbey Normal, "Past Life with Alzheimers - Spiritual Perfection - Live Spiritual Healing Gift," YouTube Video. October 18, 2016, 24:20. https://www.youtube.com/watch?v=ury42h9XRCc

does the soul gain a unique yet uncontrollable ability to exist in two worlds? Some esoteric traditions believe that the portal between the world of physicality and the world of the astral plane is located in the pineal gland. Traveling for the soul is not something new. We all travel to the astral world in our dreams—every time we go to sleep. The difference is that these toxic proteins could be linked to creating the appropriate scenario for our pineal gland to develop fault, which allows our soul to fragment its bond from our body in an uncharacteristic way. How to heal from this much physical damage is something that, to my knowledge, remains unknown.

These are the physical and spiritual reasons why we see the expression of Alzheimer's as we do. As consciousness is *the living essence of who we are*, what type of *living essence* is Alzheimer's reflecting? My answer to this question includes visions of our gigantic human party tent from chapter eleven, but this time a new factor is introduced. If the tendency of someone experiencing Alzheimer's is one where they are unconsciously trying to meet their needs through meeting the needs of others, then the fabric of connection between them and other tent poles is going to be strongly reinforced, and as we are at the end of an era, their inner closets could also be extra full. Instead of the patient retrofitting as I suggested in chapter eleven, these are souls expressing a more extreme version of polarization, perhaps one where we see ripping occurring as shifts to the structure of the party tent quicken their speed. A dynamic that creates a body living in one density and a soul that is living in another, for a time, until they fully cross over.

Epilogue

A remarkable woman named Ruth, my first energy healing teacher, would always say to us that when we decide to live a soul-centered life, that we'll have to get used to seeing only two steps in front of us, and that we'll have to learn how to be comfortable in trusting spirit with the rest. I'd like to take that wisdom even further, and say that when we live a heart-centered life, those *next two steps* become our life's fullness. You learn to live from a place where you are used to letting go of your attachments to make way for the next, *next two steps*, because you'll learn through experience that those next two steps will always come. You probably already know by now too, that if you are listening to your heart's compass, that your next two steps will be the exact right next two steps for you.

I've spent a lot of time being with the archetypal energy of the wounded inner child while writing these pages, and then for months afterward I felt those feelings in a powerful way. I held space for this big pain, and it reminded me of a moment right before I finished my school paper. The written portion was complete, but still . . . something felt unfinished. So, to help me see from a different vantage point, I decided to watch the movie *Still Alice,* a film about a woman experiencing early onset Alzheimer's disease, and when I watched the last scene I was initiated into a wailing mess of tears. As much as I had cried already, when the movie was over, I still felt like the dam to my pain had not been broken. I required a catalyst, and then felt an inner nudge to turn on the song *My Heart Will Go On* by Celine Dion. Once it was on, I kept it playing on repeat for hours. I wailed the biggest wails of heartbreak you could ever imagine—tidal waves, and I'm not exaggerating. I even had the headache to prove it. I felt what it was like to have our loved ones there, but not there as we go through the collective experience of Alzheimer's. I felt the deep pain of what that separation feels like to the human heart.

That was one year ago, and now that I've taken myself for a spin around another spiral of my own evolution, I feel the same seed, but this year's bloom comes through a more personal lens. Just like the pain of Alzheimer's comes from having our loved one there but not really there, I have felt that same experience of pain in my own heart towards myself. I became conscious of the deep pain that comes from separating our awareness from the magnificence of who we really are. It is the pain of walking away from our favorite place on earth searching for new horizons, and the longing that our soul feels when our outer being forgets about the place altogether.

***

A skill I have developed over time, is something that I like to call Shaman Vision; it's a shift in perspective (that sometimes happens naturally and spontaneously, and also initiated by conscious breath), which allows me to receive messages from the world of energy. I did this often while experiencing the isolation that Covid-19 had offered. As the world went into the first wave of the pandemic, my heart became a safe-haven for human suffering, and it came through as tones of war, sickness, and hatred—but not as we see them in the outside world around us. I held their energies in my heart, and they revealed themselves through the way in which I ate my food, and how I washed my body. They showed up in the way I cleaned my home, through what TV show I chose to watch, how I stirred the pot as I made dinner, or how I was breathing. With my shaman vision turned on, I became the witness, and I took a back seat to the energies of my programming as they ran through me. I surrendered to watching them take over and run the show for a while, and as I did, I felt like a character in a video game as something greater took governance of my body.

I felt my rib-caged heart and arms moving about the day as my body carried out its rote patterns of expression. I stayed resting in the undercurrent, and while I was there, I watched, and I learned. I see deeply through love when my shaman vision turns on, and because I was now conscious of the shadow aspects within me, my sovereign free will and the alchemical magic of my heart could claim those codes that had created my foundations and breathe them obsolete. Once presence and compassion embraced my foundations, the power of my soul could replace them with something that served my highest good. A service that is fluid in our ever-changing world.

I also let my innocence set me free. This is the part of me that does not judge, and it does me a great service because on the other side of my judgment, there is always more information. As time passed I learned to accept my programs of fear, scarcity, guilt, shame, war, hatred, and sickness at their sensational level. I felt my consciousness hugging my arms and my neck as they moved, my fingers as they spread the butter onto the toast, and my mouth as I chewed and ate my dinner in haste. I was witnessing, and I was learning, and I was seeing the truth of my nature with no need to change it whatsoever. This was the first step.

Then, just when I became friendly with my previous resistance, or less attached to my attachments, when my soul and my higher self deemed it time, I was ushered into a new phase of the process. I was invited into movement and dance, as wisps of energy had the opportunity to move through my body with the sweep of my arm and the twist of my fingers, or the shake of my thighs and the arching of my spine. With the stomping of my feet as my soles pounded the ground in gratitude, the old energy fell away to be composted by mother earth; and with the shake of my wrists and the rising of my palms up to the sky to also be evaporated by the energies of cosmic light. With loving kindness and through the tantric ecstatic nature of dance, **I released control, and surrendered to the flow of love that would heal me**. I danced the dance of love and I knew that the very same energies of conflict that run through war zones, were the same energies that run through our families. They are the same energies that run through the battleground that exists inside ourselves, right down to the individual cells that exist in the fingertip of our tiniest pinky finger. When I danced, I danced the dance of love because I knew that we all had these energies of conflict within us, *at least to some degree* because we are all human. So, I danced it through, and as I did, I said thank you and then I said NO. I said thank you because I knew that when I loved the essence of these pieces of conflict, I was healing. Then, when I pushed their expression out of my field with the force and grace of a master warrior, I was saying with my sovereignty, no—not in my sacred space. This is my birthright as a human being, and it's your birthright too.

When my dance had been danced and when the new boundaries were set, I went back to spreading the butter on toast or cleaning out the dishwasher, and in the spirit of my feminine rising, I did so as if I was making love with life. In the same way that an apple grows, a flower blooms, or in the way muffins smell when they come fresh out of the oven, I did what I was doing in a state of being in love with my experience.

For those of you who would like to grow in love, and who don't find yourself to be shamanic-ly inclined, your heart will still point you towards opportunities for growth, and you will know. Your shift could come through speaking your truth in an important relationship, or through asking for your needs to be met, and then navigating the outcomes of that asking. It could mean learning how to give your own self-approval, or learning how to let in the approval of others. It could also mean making an apology, forgiving someone for never making one, or learning to hold space for another person's perspective so that you won't have to keep making apologies. It could mean choosing to investigate the nature of your jealousy, your greed, your abandonment, your betrayal, your sadness, your gluttony, your control, or through choosing to look at a pattern you have whose outcomes are destructive.

As you advance on your journey, it could also come through a deeper dive into the nature of projection, what happens when we take ownership for our own feelings, or give others the space to make their own choices. Sometimes, there is more pain in not sharing what's buried in the closet than there is in sharing it, so finding a safe and supportive space from which to do that, and then taking yourself through the process, is what this book is all about. My beloved yoga teacher said it best, "Evolve or disappear." Pain is not something to give lip service to or to keep hiding in the closet anymore. Mother Earth no longer has space for this narrative, and loving support is available now more than ever before.

Know that your earth-suit is sacred and magnificent, and embracing this new idea is how the feminine principles will rise within you.

**

What happens when you manage to release an old belief? Or truly feel freedom from the emotional baggage you've been carrying around for so much of your life? What happens when you successfully release an old rote pattern? Well, the next part is the fun part. It is the space of the phoenix rising, of transformation, of growth, of creation, and of new beginnings. Every time you take out an old piece of your foundation, you'll be replacing it with a new one—one that hopefully serves the goodness of your essence, and one that you'll have chosen.

Once you find alignment with your soul, you will then be taught how to love yourself and your truths, and how to love your boundaries and your basic needs: mental, emotional, physical, and spiritual. If you find yourself in a place where you don't yet know what you should love about yourself, it could mean taking the time to learn who you really are, and you can start by investigating which beliefs from your family inheritance work for you and which ones don't. Do you have any repressed ambitions that have yet to be discovered? Discovery might mean doing something artistic, treating yourself to a nice dinner (just you), or starting to write in a journal.

Let your heart be the guide, and notice where your learning awaits you. Then, once the lesson of learning to love yourself is down pat, there are always next steps. You can learn how to see the needs of others, and then learn how to meet those needs without causing harm to your own core boundaries. Perhaps you will be called to learn a new ability, to create a relatable space that serves the needs of all parties, without our collective ancient traumas getting in the way any longer.

If you let your divine inner child become the one in charge of the directions (in the passenger's seat holding the road map), I think you cannot help but love yourself. It's a natural byproduct, and I wonder if you can see them now. Standing in their superhero pose with a fist to the sky, elated from the fact that you've finally found them. Tune in. Where do they want to go next? What do they want to do? What do they want to see? What makes them dance and giggle and explode with enthusiasm, and how can you channel that into your life today? Find the divine inner child who knows how to share their magic with others, and how to receive the magic of others in return. This is the part of you who is comfortable living through the heart.

***

Ask and you shall receive. Once the shift in my programming integrated into my conscious awareness, a new message came through one bright, sunny, and rhododendron-filled spring day in Vancouver. It happened after I had the simple pleasure of attending a secret yoga class at an unspecified location. We were at the end of the first wave of Covid-19, and businesses had just started opening their doors. After my first yoga class in months, I came home feeling extremely grateful. The lock clicked, the door opened, and I walked down the short hallway of my apartment to find the light pouring in through the patio doors, in the same way it did through the various plants in my living room. Its golden hues were pouring in and onto a half-knit orange scarf, which was laid out on the couch, and up and onto the shelves on the wall. These shelves were home to some books and photographs, plants, knick-knacks, and a pink peace lily that hadn't bloomed since its purchase six years prior. As I looked up, it now had a fresh bloom frolicking in the sun. I took a breath, and then I took two more.

This was a moment that called for music, so I turned on Spotify and in an inspired moment, the song that I chose was new to me. It was a song that instantly connected me to my roots called *Walk With Me* by the Celtic Women. Its fiery femininity lit me ablaze on that golden sunshine-filled day in my noisy little apartment. It's a song that helped me to consider what it would be like if all the pieces of my story, my personality, my gifts, and my wounds could be accepted, free, and able to propel me into my life's purpose. A teaching from my own loving mother then sprang forth in my mind, what would happen if I could just be a little bit kinder as I learned to see the trespasses of others as trespasses that had first been done to their own small child within. The song was sung through the voices of Celtic womanhood, while the words themselves lovingly honored the needs of our inner child and told of the joy of relating when we choose to live from a compassionate heart. They sang the medicine required for the human heart to blossom, and with as much passion and pride as an Irish and Scottish lass (meaning yours truly) has ever felt through her bones, do you have any idea of what my reaction would have been? I gather you might know me well enough by now . . . I was weeping. I was a fountain of tears, and I learned that I was ready to expand into more of who I was. I knew I had enough tools, enough strength, enough compassion, enough discipline, and enough humility to learn the next lessons. I knew I was ready.

A soul-led life, in the unique way that I experience it, bends to the winds of change, leading me to where I will learn best. So, in an ever so fast and smooth way, just like the daily dip of my toes into a rushing mountain river in springtime would feel, Vancouver's energy was leaving my feet, and in the distance I could hear the voice of my family beginning to call me home.

***

We all have a spark of God's essence within us, we all have a soul to our name, a sacred part of us that is eternal, meant to live sovereign and meant to live trauma-free. Now that you know the true fabric of your essence and the magic of your inner divine child, you can never go back to how things were. Although at times you might want to because it's the warrior and the hero's journey too. Your life might remain the same on the outside, but you've awakened to your soul, your compass on the inside is changed forever and your life's tasks experience a shift in orientation.

An activated heart will always know the next right thing to do, and so you, too, will be taught how to weave more of your soul's nature into your life in a healthy way. This is the movement of evolutionary growth that is now propelling your life forward, where your joy resides *mostly,* but sometimes it's where your sorrow and anger is too because they are all a part of mastering what it means to be human. An awakened soul is no longer a slave to the mechanisms of the matrix because it now has a greater bandwidth of awareness to make its choices from.

What that means for you and your relationships is that you first learn to be the most important person in your life (from a space of love and not ego), and then teach others to be the most important person to them. You learn how to fill your cup first, and then you can let it overflow to your spouse, your children, your neighbors, your friends, your clients, and so on. Sometimes, it means that you let others fill your cup for you too, especially in those moments when you really need it. It also means that you raise your children to know how to fill their own cup, and you can do this by mirroring back their naturalness to them. This is what helps them to create their own unique cup. To the soul, it is a position of immense honor to assist another soul to grow into all the nooks and crannies of their own earth-suit. If you are apprehensive about your position, know that your child's best self is also inborn, like how a flower blooms.

I joke about being a galactic soul sent here on a mission from outer space, and some of you might think I'm crazy for saying that. But, for everyone whom I still hold as a captive audience, it's a primer for what I'm going to say next. Just as there are control-based races in our world (who happen to be in control at the moment), there are also love and wisdom-based races too, and as our planet moves into a higher density of her expression in this new epoch, it allows these lighter psychic beings to incarnate as humans. Souls who will have more evolved spiritual gifts and ways of being; a whole cohort of beautiful, graceful, and wise souls, who need wise, warrior and heart-centered parents to raise them. That's the attunement necessary to create a reality that will foster their genius. So, if you feel a flutter in your heart as you read these words, know that you are a part of that. You can embrace how these new souls don't fit into the old matrix, instead recognize them as nature's evolutionary gift, and look to holistic, strength-building, and earth-based modalities to support their needs, as they teach us to become the salt of the earth once more.

When you wake up to a different way, no matter what age you are, you can choose to walk the path, and you can choose to walk it with grace, honor, and devotion. Then, when you've walked the path for long enough and feel ready to support those who are two steps behind you, heed that call because you too have gifts to be shared, seen, told, practiced, and experienced. As the co-creator of your reality, ask yourself, "What kind of reality do I want to live in?" and then move toward the joy of creating it.

Ask for help along the way, and seek out the people who empower you to create a reality that you would be proud to pass down to the next generation. A life led in fullness is one where you act on the things that are true to your heart, where you create them through the power of your reason and imagination, and where you take action with fire in your belly. A soul-led life requires communication with those to whom you are closest every step of the way. A soul-led life thrives in community as much as it does resting in solitude.

You can practice silencing your judgment and criticism with discerning kindness. Practice being the essence of you that is behind the masks so that you can learn to take the masks off more easily in the future. If your parents, your partners, your children, your co-workers or those in your community make mistakes, see them first as souls learning to master their own universes and have compassion *before* you have the conversations. Listen first, ask questions second, and then with more wisdom in your heart you can then take the right actions. In the end, whether this way of conscious co-creation means far-out things like we stop seeing wars, and start seeing aliens land on earth; or less far-out things like being able to share more happiness with those around us, a community who knows the power of a child's laugh, or a life where we allow the sunrise to fill us up. Whatever it is, know that you are co-creating it, and you are doing so through the programs that are encoded into your DNA.

Before we end our journey together, I want to give you official permission on behalf of your soul and Mother

Earth, to choose the feeling of goodness, innocence, and to listen to the guidance of your heart to move you forward from whatever situation you find yourself in. If it happens to be a difficult one with voices in your head, know that those voices can be silenced through love. Seek out the support you need because this is about you stepping into your birthright to feel good and alive, healthy and free, and living to your fullest potential. It is about you allowing the potent magic of your inner divine child, and the discerning power of your warrior to access and transmute whatever energies of the matrix around you that don't serve your best interest.

We all come here to this place called Earth for such unique reasons that only we can know. So, that is what I hope you'll start looking for. Learn to walk knowing only *two steps* ahead, and allow your divine inner child to lead the way. If you do this, you will change, and I am just one example of living proof. As all of this pertains to Alzheimer's, maybe I am just someone who has let her imagination go astray, and on some level I know that is actually true. However, if my arrow has flown straight, maybe our souls will have less of a reason to leave their bodies when we learn to live in a way that honors our light.

To all of you whose spark has now been lit, know that your soul's light is an *immense* gift to this world, and before you go gifting it all away, take some time to really get to know it. Remember the magnificence of who you truly are, remember it as often as you can, and from the loving heart of Doña María Apaza, "Now that we've all been blessed with a sweet heart, may we live in harmony together. May we become one heart, and walk together on one path . . . until we don't. Thank you, brothers and sisters of my heart. Come back. Come back. May the spirit return."

GLOSSARY

Astral plane—A non-physical realm where all expressions of consciousness can be experienced by the soul in a malleable way. It is said that the lowest forms of human experiences and the highest forms (both heaven and hell), can be lived out in this realm.

Attunement—The ability to allow our internal state to resonate with the internal state of another, in order to better understand, support, and relate to them.

β-amyloid plaques—The beta-amyloid protein involved in Alzheimer's comes in several different molecular forms that collect between neurons. It is formed from the breakdown of a larger protein, called amyloid precursor protein. One form, beta-amyloid 42, is thought to be especially toxic. In the Alzheimer's brain, abnormal levels of this naturally occurring protein clump together to form plaques that collect between neurons and disrupt cell function.[1]

Channel—Someone who can carry or deliver information from one density of consciousness to another. Channeling is when a human being allows the energy of a non-physical being to borrow their body to share a message with earth.

Claircognizance—The ability to *just know* information, which often offers a clear sense of the truth in the moment.

---

[1]   "What Happens to the Brain in Alzheimer's Disease?" National Institute on Aging (website), last reviewed May 16, 2017, https://www.nia.nih.gov/health/what-happens-brain-alzheimers-disease.

Co-creative—Co-creation happens naturally when we consider the other (person, animal, spirit, crystal, flower, or any other form of living being) who we are creating with as equal to us. When we come to situations in a state of presence, honoring equality (in essence) first, and inequality (in skill and offering) second, we catalyze creation in a powerful way because *two is better than one.*

Core boundaries—Personal boundaries are guidelines, rules, or limits that a person creates to identify reasonable, safe, and permissible ways for other people to behave towards them. In living relationships, the boundaries of a healthy ego will be flexible and malleable, which means that many of our boundaries will be changeable moment to moment. Core boundaries are the deeper foundations of us that are not changeable; some will be unique to each person, while many are inherent to our basic human rights.

Co-regulation—The precursor to self-regulating the energies we receive from the world. The auric fields of children are focused on growing their emotional (energy in motion) processing foundations from ages two to seven, and it's here they require an adult to help co-regulate their emotions with them. At the root of this process is the adult's ability to hold space for the emotion that is being integrated in a space of presence, themselves.

1. Label: teach the use of words to express emotions.
2. Model: show waiting and self-calming strategies.
3. Redirect: divert the child's attention to a regulating behavior.
4. Support: provide a warm, nurturing, and supportive relationship.
5. Positive: use positive reinforcement when rules are followed.
6. Clear: set and maintain clear expectations and limits.

Dantian point—This term originates from China. There are three dantian points in the body, and the one I am speaking to is the lower dantian point. While the chakras are spinning vortexes of energy that protrude from the body, the dantian is a nerve plexus of energy inside the body roughly five milimeters in diameter and grows stronger with practice. The lower dantian is located a few fingers below the navel and inside the sacral chakra. It houses your vital energy, power, and essence.

Dogma—Information that is passed down to us in a way that does not cultivate the uniqueness and power of our essence, and which is most influential in childhood during a time when the power to integrate that information as conscious co-creators in the present moment is not available to us.

Ego—The ego is another word for the individuated nature of our incarnation, and it includes all aspects of us that form our individuality. The ego is innate, and neither negative nor positive. In a healthy state, it should be experienced as malleable and centralized.

Eros—Eros is one of the four ancient Greek terms that can be rendered in English as *love*. The other three are storge, philia, and agape. Eros refers to passionate love or romance, and it's an energetic signature that is activated in adolescence. From another vantage point, it is also how we can feel a higher love for ourselves through the other, and it's reflective of embodied divinity in human form.

Fawn—In the context of trauma, is when we respond to a threat by hyperfocusing on meeting the needs of that which is making us feel threatened.

Fifth density—This is the density of the golden age. Manifestation happens almost instantly here, and so we need training before we graduate to this way of being. It is where love, personal sovereignty, truth, and a connection to our universal community is realized.

Flower essence—Flower essences were thought to have been used by various civilizations for centuries, most commonly as dew collected from flowers in the early morning. Essences are usually held in water or brandy.

Fourth density—Is the density of reality that acts as a bridge to the fifth density. Once we wake up spiritually, and we realize that we are the creators of our reality, it is the density where we can take personal responsibility and correct course, it allows our consciousness to slow down so that we can look at our programs. It is a space of witness where we can choose new thoughts, process our old emotions, and create new future pathways of expression. Sometimes the fourth density is interchangeable with the term astral plane.

Higher self—Typically considered the part of us who is more connected to source or God, and the part of us we can look to when seeking guidance. In the energy field, the higher version of us in this lifetime is connected to our fifth layer and fifth density self.

Hold space—A person holding space is creating a dynamic of non-judgment, where it is safe for those they are holding space for to be mentally, emotionally, physically, and spiritually authentic (while the boundaries of the space holder also remain intact). It could be considered a feminine principle, and a way of being that is activated through presence.

"I release control, and surrender to the flow of love that will heal me"—These are lyrics from a song called *I Release Control* by Alexa Sunshine Rose. If you are curious, look it up online, close your eyes, dance or be still, receive and let the healing happen.

Karma—The energetic data held in our subconscious from our soul's experiences that have yet to be reconciled or integrated. The karma from our previous actions as a soul can be both negative and positive, and will affect how we experience life in the present moment if balance through awareness and lesson learning has yet to happen.

Natural law—There are thirteen principles of natural law: mentalism, correspondence, polarity, rhythm, suggestion, response, cause and effect, transformation, transcendence, verification, cycles, vibration, and gender. When we live in truth and harmony with ourselves and others, we are living in truth and harmony within the Universal Natural Laws. This way of living drastically increases the quality of life on earth for everyone. (Paraphrased from goldenageofgaia.com)

Meridian lines—The Chinese equivalent of *nadis*.

Nadis—The ayurvedic word for light pathways in the physical body that connect to the chakras and that move and flow life force or prana.

Neurofibrillary tangles—Neurofibrillary tangles are abnormal accumulations of a protein called tau that collect inside neurons. Healthy neurons, in part, are supported internally by structures called microtubules, which help guide nutrients and molecules from the cell body to the axon and dendrites. In healthy neurons, tau normally binds to and stabilizes microtubules. In Alzheimer's disease, however, abnormal chemical changes cause tau to detach from microtubules and stick to other tau molecules, forming threads that eventually join to form tangles inside neurons. These tangles block the neuron's transport system, which harms the synaptic communication between neurons.[2]

Prana—The Sanskrit word for lifeforce energy or life breath. Prana means breathing forth, and is based on the idea that vital or life force energy is always dynamic.

Projection—Happens in the energy field when we can not yet hold the program we are running in the state of the witness, or in presence. When the trauma-based programs that we have are still unconscious to us, we will naturally project the stories and emotions they hold on to the people who are closest to us while in a state of fight, flight, freeze, or fawn. Consider the outermost layer of your auric field as a screen, and our programs as the plot line. The positive side of projection is that it allows us to see the stories we hold, which is the first step to deconstructing them.

Relational cords—The official energetic term for the lines of energy that connect us to other people and that hold the expectations, ways of responding, power dynamics, and so on. When these cords are created unconsciously, they will often run on autopilot. When we desire the evolution or release of relationship dynamics as we grow, it's helpful to access the location of these cords in the energy field as we do.

---

2   "What Happens to the Brain in Alzheimer's Disease?" National Institute on Aging (website), last reviewed May 16, 2017, https://www.nia.nih.gov/health/what-happens-brain-alzheimers-disease.

Soul contracts—With the assistance of our spirit guides, these are the binding agreements we make pre-incarnation related to the lessons we wish to learn, the tasks we wish to complete, and the other souls we consent to meet along the way who will help us in completing our lessons.

Spirit guides—The entourage of non-physical beings who have signed love-based contracts to support you in this lifetime. They could be ancestors, earth spirits, angels, and higher dimensional souls, as there are many hierarchies and kingdoms of expression before we reach the experience of non-separation with source consciousness.

Stacking—When we live unaware of the power of our emotions, and are running unconscious and trauma-based relational programs, these different densities of energy in motion will stack and condense in our emotional body. Excavating programs may include processing many layers of emotions (check out the emotional guidance scale, available online), and many layers of past experience. These scenarios may appear different on the surface, but are running on the same root program (usually created in childhood).

Third density—The version of reality that our current mass collective consciousness lives in. It is one where it seems that the physical world is the only thing that is real. It is a world of polarity and separation.

Transmute—To change in form, nature, or substance. In the realm of human energetics, transmutation is a natural function of a soul-centered heart. Here is how you do that:

1. Become aware of the energetic programs you are running.

2. Explore these programs through the loving embrace of compassion.
3. Explore and envision a new solution that is supported by your higher self.
4. Create change through action. You have become a successful transmuter of energies!

Triggers—Any phrase, action, object, emotion, smell, touch (at the root a vibrational signature) that causes you to recreate or relive your original traumatic experience. Triggers bring you out of presence and reconnect you with your original, unprocessed energetic program.

Warriors of the rainbow prophecy (bonus definition)—An oral prophecy passed down through many indigenous cultures depicting a time on earth where its children would come together in love and unity, and unite as all colors of the rainbow. It will be a time of peace, remembrance, and harmony upon earth.

Window of tolerance—A term coined by Dr. Dan Seigel to describe the bandwidth of energy in motion that we are able to experience in a state of presence. Our optimal zone of arousal, where we are able to manage and thrive.

ADDITIONAL RESOURCES

ENERGY HEALING AND HUMAN ENERGETICS

Kala Ambrose, *The Awakened Aura: Experiencing the Evolution of Your Energy Body*. Woodbury: Llewellyn Worldwide, 2011.

Barbara Ann Brennan, *Light Emerging: The Journey of Personal Healing*. Toronto: Bantam Books, 1993.

Cyndi Dale, *The Complete Book of Chakra Healing: Activate the Transformative Power of Your Energy Centers*. Woodbury: Llewellyn Publications, 2009.

Donna Eden and David Feinstein, *Energy Medicine*. New York: Tarcher/Putnam, 1999.

Anodea Judith, *Eastern Body, Western Mind Psychology and the Chakra System as a Path to the Self*. Kolkata: Alchemy, 2006.

Nirmal Lumpkin and Japa Kaur Khalsa, *Enlightened Bodies: Exploring Physical and Subtle Human Anatomy*. Santa Cruz: Kundalini Research Institute, 2015.

Caroline Myss, *Anatomy of the Spirit: The Seven Stages of Power and Healing*. New York: Harmony Books, 2017.

Caroline Myss, *Sacred Contracts: Awakening Your Divine Potential*. London: Transworld Digital, 2010.

James L Oschman, *Energy Medicine: The Scientific Basis* Edinburgh: Elsevier, 2016.

PLANT MEDICINE

Carole Guyett, *Sacred Plant Initiations: Communicating with Plants for Healing and Higher Consciousness*. Rochester: Bear & Company, 2015.

Rachel Harris, *Listening to Ayahuasca: New Hope for Depression, Addiction, PTSD, and Anxiety*. Novato: New World Library, 2017.

Jonathon Miller Weisberger, *Rainforest Medicine*. New York: Random House USA, 2013.

SELF-LOVE

Teal Swan, *Shadows Before Dawn: Finding the Light of Self-Love Through Your Darkest Times*. Carlsbad, CA: Hay House, 2015.

SPIRITUAL AWAKENING

Melody Lynn Beattie, *Finding Your Way Home: A Soul Survival Kit*. New York: HarperCollins, 1998.

Richard Rudd, *Gene Keys: Unlocking the Higher Purpose Hidden in Your DNA*. London: Watkins, 2015.

Don Miguel Ruiz, *The Four Agreements*. Thorndike: Amber-Allen Publishing, 1997.

Leslie Temple-Thurston and Brad Laughlin, *The Marriage of Spirit*. Cork: Book Baby, 2000.

Leslie Temple-Thurston, *Returning to Oneness: the Seven Keys of Ascension*. Cork: BookBaby, 2002.

SPIRITUALITY AND ALZHEIMER'S

Megan Carnarius, *A Deeper Perspective on Alzheimer's and Other Dementias: Practical Tools with Spiritual Insights*. Forres: Findhorn Press, 2015.

Maggie La Tourelle, *The Gift of Alzheimer's: Heart & Soul Journey*. New York: HarperCollins, 2014.

TRAUMA

Ron Kurtz and Hector Prestera, *The Body Reveals: How to Read Your Own Body*. San Francisco: Harper & Row, 1984.

Bessel Van der Kolk, *The Body Keeps the Score: Brain, Mind, and Body in the Healing of Trauma*. New York: Penguin Books, 2015.

Acknowledgments

If it wasn't for the cherished friends and co-creators who embraced me on this journey, I wouldn't be a published author. Thank you to my beloved family; my father for his investment in this project, my mother for her gentle embrace of my vision, my sister Erin for being my cheerleader and for protecting my voice, and my sister Cassie for loving me with a kind heart and an open ear. You guys are the absolute best.

Thank you to GBR, my publishers, for being so accommodating with the ever-evolving manuscript (and timeline), to Angelica my editor for believing in the message, and to my teacher Ruth for empowering my *Sparks From the Heart* journey through to the finish line.

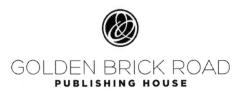

GOLDEN BRICK ROAD
PUBLISHING HOUSE

Link arms with us as we pave new paths to a better a more expansive world.

Golden Brick Road Publishing House (GBRPH) is a small, independently initiated boutique press created to provide social-innovation entrepreneurs, experts, and leaders a space in which they can develop their writing skills and content to reach existing audiences as well as new readers.

Serving an ambitious catalogue of books by individual authors, GBRPH also boasts a unique co-author program that capitalizes on the concept of "many hands make light work." GBRPH works with our authors as partners. Thanks to the value, originality, and fresh ideas we provide our readers, GBRPH books have won eighteen awards and are available in bookstores across the world.

We aim to develop content that effects positive social change while empowering and educating our members to help them strengthen themselves and the services they provide to their clients.

Iconoclastic, ambitious, and set to enable social innovation, GBRPH is helping our writers/partners make cultural change one book at a time.

Inquire today at www.goldenbrickroad.pub